PSYCHIATRIC CONSEQUENCES OF BRAIN DISEASE IN THE ELDERLY

A Focus on MANAGEMENT

PSYCHIATRIC CONSEQUENCES OF BRAIN DISEASE IN THE ELDERLY

A Focus on
MANAGEMENT

Edited by
David K. Conn
*Baycrest Centre for Geriatric Care
and University of Toronto
Toronto, Ontario, Canada*

Adrian Grek
*Queen Street Mental Health Centre
and University of Toronto
Toronto, Ontario, Canada*

and
Joel Sadavoy
*Baycrest Centre for Geriatric Care
and University of Toronto
Toronto, Ontario, Canada*

PLENUM PRESS • NEW YORK AND LONDON

Library of Congress Cataloging in Publication Data

Psychiatric consequences of brain disease in the elderly: a focus on mangement /
edited by David K. Conn, Adrian Grek, and Joel Sadavoy.
    p.   cm.
Based on a symposium held May 29, 1987 in Toronto, Ont., Canada.
Includes bibliographies and index.
ISBN 0-306-43216-1
    1. Geriatric neuropsychiatry—Congresses. 2. Brain—Aging—Congresses. 3. Brain
—Diseases—Complications and sequelae—Congresses. I. Conn, David K. II. Grek,
Adrian. III. Sadavoy, Joel, 1945-
    [DNLM: 1. Mental Disorders—in old age—congresses. 2. Mental Disorders—
therapy—congresses. WT 150 P974 1987]
RC451.4.A5P75   1989
618.97'689—dc20
DNLM/DLC   89-8434
for Library of Congress   CIP

Based on proceedings of a symposium entitled
Psychiatric Consequences of Brain Disease in the Elderly:
A Focus on Management, held May 29, 1987,
in Toronto, Ontario, Canada

© 1989 Plenum Press, New York
A Division of Plenum Publishing Corporation
233 Spring Street, New York, N.Y. 10013

Printed in the United States of America

TO OUR WIVES AND CHILDREN

CONTRIBUTORS

Graham Berman, M.B., Ch.B., F.R.C.P.(C)
Staff Psychiatrist, Baycrest Centre for Geriatric Care
Assistant Professor, Department of Psychiatry, University of Toronto
Training Analyst, Toronto Institute of Psychoanalysis, Toronto, Ontario

Gene D. Cohen, M.D., Ph.D.
Director of the Program on Aging at the National Institute of Mental
Health
Clinical Professor of Psychiatry, Georgetown University School of
Medicine, Washington, D.C.

David K. Conn, M.B., B.Ch., F.R.C.P.(C)
Coordinator, Consultation-Liaison Psychiatry Service, Baycrest Centre for
Geriatric Care
Assistant Professor, Department of Psychiatry, University of Toronto,
Toronto, Ontario

Jeffrey L. Cummings, M.D.
Director of the Neurobehaviour Unit, West Los Angeles Veterans
Administration Medical Center
Associate Professor of Neurology and of Psychiatry and Biobehavioural
Science, UCLA School of Medicine, Los Angeles, California

Adrian Grek, M.B., B.Ch., F.R.C.P.(C)
Chief, Psychogeriatric Service, Queen Street Mental Health Centre
Assistant Professor, Department of Psychiatry, University of Toronto,
Toronto, Ontario

Guy-Bernard Proulx, Ph.D.
Director, Department of Psychology, Baycrest Centre for Geriatric Care,
Toronto, Ontario

Anne Robinson, R.N.
Nurse Clinician, Department of Psychiatry, Baycrest Centre for Geriatric
Care, Toronto, Ontario

Joel Sadavoy, M.D., F.R.C.P.(C)
Head, Department of Psychiatry, Baycrest Centre for Geriatric Care
Associate Professor, Department of Psychiatry, University of Toronto
Toronto, Ontario

Stuart A. Schneck, M.D.
Professor of Neurology and Pathology (Neuropathology) and Associate Dean
for Clinical Affairs, University of Colorado School of Medicine, Denver,
Colorado

Kenneth Shulman, M.D., F.R.C.P.(C)
Head, Division of Geriatric Psychiatry, Sunnybrook Medical Centre
Interim Director, Division of Geriatrics, Faculty of Medicine and
Coordinator, Division of Geriatrics, Department of Psychiatry, University
of Toronto, Toronto, Ontario

Sheldon S. Tobin, Ph.D.
Director of the Ringel Institute of Gerontology and Professor in the
School of Social Welfare, State University of New York at Albany

PREFACE

Alzheimer's disease, stroke and Parkinson's disease are the most prevalent brain diseases in the elderly. The psychiatric and behavioural consequences of these and other brain disorders contribute greatly to the decline in function of these patients, often leading to greater suffering and a decreased quality of life, placement in institutions and increased stress on the family and other caregivers. The authors in this book discuss the psychiatric consequences of brain disease in the elderly with a particular focus on the *management* of these disorders.

We have tried to keep the content of this book clinically relevant throughout by using a series of case examples and by emphasizing the various treatment strategies and forms of management available to the health care professional. In attempting to understand these disorders, it is important to place equal emphasis on biological, psychological and social factors. Because of the complexity and chronicity of these conditions, multidisciplinary intervention is crucial. We believe that this book will be helpful to all those working with the elderly, whether in the community or in the institution. This includes physicians, nurses, social workers, occupational therapists, psychologists and all those working with this patient population.

The initial planning and development of this book resulted from a Symposium entitled "Psychiatric Consequences of Brain Disease in the Elderly: A Focus on Management" which was presented in Toronto, Ontario, Canada on the 29th of May, 1987 by the Department of Psychiatry, Baycrest Centre for Geriatric Care and the Division of Geriatric Psychiatry of the University of Toronto. This symposium brought together a panel of international speakers to discuss specific approaches to the management of neuropsychiatric disorders in the elderly.

The case vignettes in this book bring life and added meaning to the subject and form a bridge between theory and actual clinical problems. Our understanding of these issues often stems from the special and deep relationship which develops between professionals and their patients. As clinicians we must be aware of our indebtedness to our patients and their families, as we search together for an understanding of how to cope with these often insurmountable problems.

We hope that this book will stimulate and guide the reader to consider the variety of possible interventions in the care of these patients and to understand that the most effective treatment may involve the employment of several of these approaches. This may help to keep the wolf of nihilism away from our door.

David Conn
Adrian Grek
Joel Sadavoy

ACKNOWLEDGEMENTS

We would like to thank Mrs. Paula Ferreira for her great patience, hard work and diligence in the preparation of the manuscript and Ms. Malerie Feldman for her ongoing help and encouragement. We would also like to thank Ms. Pat Vann and Ms. Melanie Yelity at Plenum for their support and helpful advice. We would like to acknowledge the excellent efforts of Mr. John Conner (Illustration) and Mr. Simon Tanenbaum (Design), who prepared the book cover. We would like to thank our colleagues, who have contributed to this volume, for their cooperation and enthusiasm. Finally we are indebted to the administrative and clinical staff of Baycrest Centre for Geriatric Care for their continuing support and for their encouragement with regard to this publication.

CONTENTS

CHAPTER 1

NEUROPSYCHIATRIC SYNDROMES IN THE ELDERLY:

AN OVERVIEW

David K. Conn, M.B., B.Ch., F.R.C.P.(C)
Baycrest Centre for Geriatric Care
University of Toronto
Toronto, Ontario

"Dementia, by separating and isolating certain faculties, and by
interfering with the outcome of mind, enables one to get a clearer
view of mind than is to be gleaned from the study of the normal mind
in healthy action." George H. Savage, (Physician and superintendent
of Bethlem Royal Hospital) 1890.

Neuropsychiatric syndromes may be defined as the clusters of
behaviour, mood, emotional and cognitive disturbance which occur as the
result of brain disease. The organic mental disorders, as defined in the
DSM-III-R, (American Psychiatric Association, 1987) can be used to
classify this group of syndromes. Neuropsychiatry has been described as
"the specialty dealing with both organic and functional diseases of the
nervous system" (Stedman's Medical Dictionary, 1982). However, in trying
to conceptualize neuropsychiatric disease, the artificial division of
disorders into "organic" and "functional" seems redundant. A more
integrated view, linking physiological and mental processes, is required.
Fortunately, there has been a dramatic growth in interest and research in
this field with major contributions from geriatric and biological
psychiatry, behavioural neurology and neuropsychology.

Neuropsychiatric disorders are responsible for a disproportionate
burden on the health care system. This arises, in part, from the enormous
growth in the geriatric population. The *world* population over age
60 increased from 200 million in 1950 to 350 million in 1975 and is
projected to be 1.1 billion in 2025. (Lowy, 1986). The percentage of
people over age 60 will be 13.7% as compared to 8.5% in 1975. The
percentage of persons over age 80 will rise proportionally higher than the
rest of the 60+ group. In the United States in 1900 only 4% of the total
population was over 65. As of 1975, 10% (22.4 million) was in this

1

group. In 1982 they reached 11.6%. By the year 2000, 35 million Americans will exceed age 65 (13.1% of the population) and by the year 2050 there will be 67 million older Americans (21.7% of the population) (Lowy, 1986). The relevance of these figures to neuropsychiatric disorders becomes evident when considered together with epidemiological data. The United States National Centre for Health Statistics (1979) revealed that approximately 20% of all nursing home residents (250,000) had a mental disorder (i.e. psychiatric illness or dementia) as their *primary* source of disability and that nearly 70% (more than 900,000 residents) had a chronic mental disorder contributing to social dependency, functional impairment and a need for long-term care. The annual cost of caring for patients with dementia in 1978 was $12 billion and the projected cost, by the year 2030, is $30 billion (in 1978 value dollars) (Plum, 1979).

Clearly, as the incidence of these diseases increases, the costs will continue to escalate. However, the cost in human suffering for patients and their families cannot be measured. There will be growing pressure on our medical and social systems, and careful planning and organization of services will be required. The demands on long-term care and community resources for the elderly are going to increase at a dramatic rate. Judging from the current length of waiting lists it appears that the system already may be failing.

One group of patients which is especially likely to contribute greatly to the escalating needs for health care is the elderly with brain disease. Lishman (1978) classifies the causes of organic brain disorders into 11 groups, as follows: 1. Degenerative (including senile dementia, Alzheimer's disease, Pick's disease, Huntington's disease, Parkinson's disease), 2. Space-occupying lesions, 3. Trauma, 4. Infection, 5. Vascular Pathology, 6. Epilepsy, 7. Metabolic disorders, 8. Endocrine disorders, 9. Toxicity, 10. Anoxia, and 11. Vitamin deficiencies. The most prevalent brain diseases in the elderly are the dementias, especially Alzheimer's disease and multi-infarct dementia, stroke, and the various forms of parkinsonism. Of these, it is clear that the dementias constitute the greatest public health problem. It appears that 1.3-6.2% of all individuals over age 65 suffer from dementia, with milder impairment in 2.6-15.4% (Mortimer, Schuman and French, 1981). These percentages increase dramatically in the population over age 80, with annual *incidence* rates of up to 2.5% (Hagnell, Lanke, Porsman, Ohman and Ojesjo, 1983).

Henderson (1987) cites four reasons why Alzheimer's disease is such a serious problem. They include the remarkable demographic shift as discussed above, the age-specific incidence rate and its chronicity, the fact that most individuals with Alzheimer's disease live in the community and that the disorder is of unknown etiology.

MODELS OF DISEASE

A variety of models have been proposed in an attempt to explain the complex behavioural manifestations of neuropsychiatric disorders all of which have a certain validity and usefulness. Some models describe a simple relationship between anatomical-pathological change and behavioural abnormalities, while others focus on neurophysiological, neurochemical, neuropharmacological, psychodynamic, behavioural, and sociological views of these disorders. However, there is an obvious danger of employing too narrow a model of care. For example, in a clinical setting, if the treatment team believes that a patient's depression is solely related to the destruction of certain neurons in a discrete part of the brain and that the only treatment required is an anti-depressant medication, this may result in the neglect of a variety of psychological, social and environmental treatment options. Conversely, if depression occurring in a medically ill patient is regarded simply as an understandable "psychological reaction" then potentially crucial psychopharmacological treatment may not be prescribed.

More comprehensive models of illness are integrated and avoid these dicotomies, for example the biopsychosocial model prosposed by Engel (1977). The illness behaviour model which can be seen in figure 1, incorporates an integrated biopsychosocial model with an attempt to also understand the behavioural manifestations of the disorder, including health seeking behaviour (McHugh and Vallis, 1986). Comprehensive models, such as the illness behaviour model, while useful for conceptualizing the patient's problem and possible management approaches, are often so complex that it is extremely difficult, given our current state of knowledge, to study them empirically. It may be necessary to break down the components of the puzzle into smaller parts in order to scientifically study certain aspects of these disorders. Psychodynamic, behavioural and sociological components are discussed in later chapters. The balance of this chapter will focus on the relationship between behaviour and biological aspects of brain function and describe the classification of neuropsychiatric disorders and psychiatric consequences of specific neurological diseases.

NEUROANATOMY

The careful study of patients with localized brain lesions has been the basis of our knowledge about the relationship between brain anatomy and behaviour. Knowledge in this field has particularly accelerated since the arrival of new, sophisticated, brain-scanning devices such as Computerized Tomography (CT), Positron-Emission Tomography (PET) and Nuclear Magnetic Resonance (NMR).

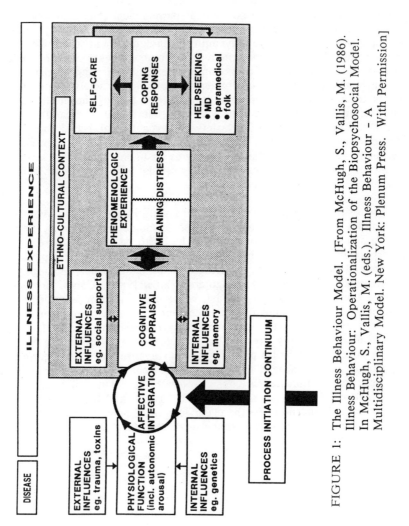

FIGURE 1: The Illness Behaviour Model. [From McHugh, S., Vallis, M. (1986). Illness Behaviour: Operationalization of the Biopsychosocial Model. In McHugh, S., Vallis, M. (eds.). Illness Behaviour - A Multidisciplinary Model. New York: Plenum Press. With Permission]

There is much debate about the degree of anatomical specialization within the brain. Clearly the amount of tissue destroyed, the location of the lesion in the brain and the nature of the disease process itself will all determine, to some extent, the manifestations of a particular brain disorder. The original debate involved Lashley (1929) who proposed that all areas of the brain were of equal importance in intellectual functioning and that the critical factor was the total amount of brain tissue destroyed rather than the exact location of the lesion. Other neurologists felt that there was a more clear-cut relationship between structure and function and attempted to identify particular anatomical areas which were associated with definite changes in function. Chapman and Wolff (1959) studied the relationship between the amount of tissue removed during the surgical excision of a brain tumour and post-operative intellectual impairment. They found that even when brain destruction was not extensive, that is involving less than 120 grams of tissue, there were still changes in adaptive capacities. They described four categories of such symptoms; 1. changes in the expression of needs, appetites and drives, 2. altered capacity to adapt for the achievement of goals (with decreased anticipation, planning, arranging, inventing, modulating, and discriminating), 3. decreased integration of socially appropriate reactions of defense and distress and 4. decreased capacity to recover from the effects of stress.

It appears that although anatomical specialization clearly exists in the human brain, lesion location alone is not sufficient to explain certain psychological and behavioural abnormalities. Lishman (1978) uses the term "regional affiliations" and states that "what we ask of psychological symptoms as guides to formal pathology must be considerably less than we expect of neurological signs" (p. 29). He suggests caution in trying to link emotional, motivational or personality abnormalities to specific, localized brain pathology and notes that psychotic symptoms in particular have alluded ties to focal brain pathology.

Frontal Lobe Sydromes

The syndromes which result from damage to the frontal lobes are particularly striking. Three frontal lobe syndromes are described, although, in clinical practice, they generally overlap. These syndromes include the orbito-frontal syndrome characterized by disinhibition and impulsive behaviour; the frontal convexity syndrome in which apathy is the predominant problem; and the medial-frontal syndrome associated with akinesia (Cummings, 1985).

The most dramatic behavioural abnormalities are related to disinhibition which may lead to a total change in an individual's personality. There is loss of social tact, tastelessness and inappropriate speech and there may be anti-social acts. Irritable and labile emotions may develop with periodic euphoria, inappropriate jocularity (Witzelsucht), hyperactivity or hypomanic behaviour. There may be inappropriate sexual disinhibition and preoccupations. Cognitive impairment may be very subtle and difficult to establish. The individual is often distractable and there is lack of vigilence with regard to the capacity to evaluate their own behaviour and performance. Behaviour is often impulsive with decreased insight and judgement.

On clinical examination there is often apathy or psychomotor retardation. The patient may demonstrate an inability to program novel motor activity and to use verbal functions to guide such activities, leading to perseveration or motor impersistence. Decreased word fluency, abstraction and categorization skills, impairment on tests of abstract reasoning and difficulty shifting set (e.g. Wisconsin card sorting test) are also common. The differential diagnosis of the causes of frontal lobe syndromes includes trauma, external compressive neoplasms (meningiomas), intrinsic tumours (gliomas), degenerative and demyelinating diseases and hydrocephalus. Among the dementias Alzheimer's disease is more likely to involve the frontal convexity region, whereas Pick's disease more often affects the orbito-frontal cortex.

Limbic System

The limbic system is the ring of gray matter and tracts bordering the hemispheres in the medial portions of the brain, which appears to play an important role in emotions. From a phylogenetic point of view, parts of the limbic system are among the oldest portions of the cortex. The limbic system has been described as "a meeting place for the disciplines of psychiatry and neurology" and "more of a philosophic concept than a discreet anatomical or physiological system..." (Pincus and Tucker, 1978, pg. 58).

Papez (1937) first pointed out the possible relation between the limbic system and emotion, behaviour and visceral reactivity. He believed that the hippocampus was an important regulator of emotions via the hypothalamic centres. He predicted that, following stimulation of the hippocampus, there would be prolonged, active, electrical discharges that essentially would remain within the limbic system without spread to the neo-cortical areas. He further predicted that such "reverberating circuits" would produce marked changes in the subjective emotional life of an individual.

Figure 2 represents the major anatomical structures and pathways within the limbic system. There are at least four major fibrous pathways within the limbic system (Strub and Black, 1981). The first pathway is

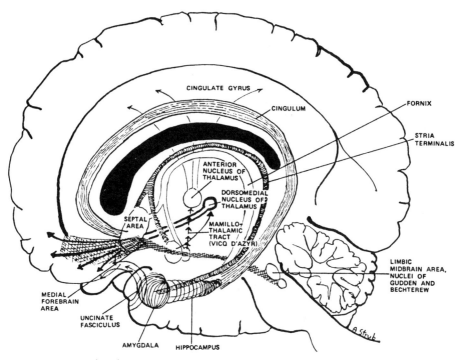

FIGURE 2: Limbic Structures. [From Strub, R.L., Black, F.W. (1981). Organic Brain Sydromes - An Introduction to Neuro-behavioural Disorders. Philadelphia: F.A. Davis Company. With Permission.]

the fornix whose fibres originate in the hippocampus and terminate in the mamillary bodies and in the septal nuclei. The second pathway is the mamillo-thalamic tract of Vicq d'Azyr. The third pathway is the stria terminalis which connects the amygdala to the ventromedial hypothalamus and the septal region. The fourth major pathway is the medial forebrain bundle which originates in the inferior frontal cortex and septal nuclei and, passing through the lateral hypothalamus, continues to the limbic mid-brain area.

The limbic system appears to be a particularly crucial modulator of instinctual behaviour. These instincts, which are found in all animals and are related to self-preservation and perpetuation of the species, include eating, fighting, fear and sexual desire. It should be stressed, of course, that the limbic system does not operate in isolation and that there is close interaction with the ascending arousal system, the basal ganglia and the neocortex.

Feeding instincts are primarily controlled by the hypothalamus. Excessive feeding can be induced in animals by stimulation of the lateral hypothalamus or destruction of the ventromedial hypothalamic nuclei (Strub and Black, 1981). Patients with lesions in the ventromedial zone demonstrate marked hyperphagia (Reeves and Plum, 1969) whereas patients with ventrolateral damage become anorexic and emaciated.

Aggression and the ability to know when to escape danger (flight) are crucial survival instincts. They appear to be controlled by the temporal limbic lobe, amygdala and hippocampus. Klüver and Bucy (1939) discovered that vicious monkeys were reformed to docility by bilateral removal of their temporal lobes. Stimulation of the amygdala or hippocampus often causes violent attack behaviour. Aggressive or violent behaviour has been occasionally described in patients with temporal lobe epilepsy. Aggression has also been reported in patients with destructive lesions in the ventromedial hypothalamus.

Sexuality and mating behaviour, while clearly involving higher cortical control in man, appear to be subserved in part, by the septal nuclei and the anterior cingulate gyri. The septal nuclei have been referred to as the pleasure centre of man because subjects will repeatedly stimulate this part of the brain without other external reinforcement (Jacques, 1979). In one female patient with marked hypersexuality, a tumour in the anterior cingulate gyrus was discovered (Erikson, 1945). The temporal lobes may have an inhibitory influence upon sexual behaviour. Hyposexuality has been described in patients with temporal lobe epilepsy.

Of critical relevance is the fact that memory appears to be intimately related to several limbic structures. It has been shown that bilateral damage to the hippocampi significantly impairs the ability to learn. The mamillary bodies and dorsal medial thalami are also of vital importance for the processing, storage and retrieval of memory.

The Cortex

Knowledge about the relationship between the anatomy of the cortex, its various areas as described by Brodmann and their associated functions is growing. We have begun to understand which parts of the cortex subserve motor behaviour and sensory input and the complex association areas in which information from various sensory inputs is integrated. Language function, in particular, has been studied extensively and in the majority of the population i.e. the right-handed population and some left-handed individuals the left hemisphere is clearly dominant for language functions. The areas subserving the major processes of language, that is, comprehension of spoken language, verbal reasoning, production of speech, reading and writing have been delineated. The relationship between cerebral laterality and psychiatric illness and "the lateralization of emotion" has become the focus of interesting investigation. The findings suggest distinct differences in the functioning of the two hemispheres (Wexler, 1980).

Higher intellectual functioning includes verbal reasoning, creative thinking, complex visual-spatial tasks and highly skilled motor actions. This may require complex interactions and synthesis of stored language, visual memories and tactile images. It is believed that these higher-order intellectual functions are possible because of the rich association areas in the postrolandic cortex and that most complex intellectual processes are carried out in these regions.

NEUROCHEMISTRY

Figure 3 shows the distribution of the major neuro-transmitter systems of the brain. Our knowledge of the neurochemical abnormalities in such diseases as Parkinson's, Alzheimer's, and Huntington's diseases has grown dramatically and offers hope of new psychopharmacological advances in treatment. This occurs in parallel to our increased understanding of the underlying neurotransmitter abnormalities in various psychiatric disorders such as schizophrenia and endogenous depression. Although our knowledge in this area is relatively limited, it clearly adds tremendous potential to our understanding of the relationship between behavioural changes and underlying brain abnormalities. For example, in idiopathic Parkinson's disease, the outstanding defect appears to be degeneration of brain stem neurons which produce dopamine and norepinephrine (Lishman, 1987). Normally dopamine is found in high concentration in pigmented cells of the substantia nigra, the nigro-striatal tract and its terminals in the caudate and putamen. It is now clearly established that dopamine levels are dramatically reduced in the brains of most patients with Parkinson's disease. Evidently, alterations in the dopamine-acetylcholine balance leading to cholinergic dominance in the striatum causes parkinsonism. Other neuro-transmitters may be implicated as well. Concentrations of norepinephrine and serotonin are also reduced. *Other* dopaminergic pathways may also be impaired such as the mesolimbic pathway. This is believed to be particularly relevant to some of the psychiatric complications of Parkinson's disease.

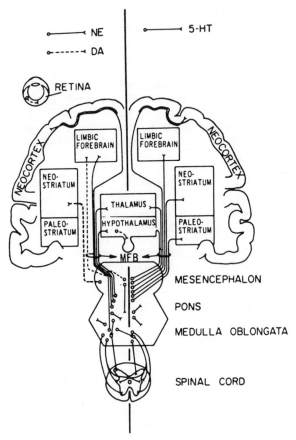

FIGURE 3: Diagram showing the distribution of the major neuro-transmitter
systems of the brain. Reproduced from Anden, N.E., Dahlstrom,
A., Fuxe, K., Larsson, K., Olson, L., Ungerstedt, U. Ascending
monoamine neurons to the diencephalon. Acta Physiol Scand.,
1966, 67 Fig.10. With Permission.

NEUROENDOCRINE RESPONSE

Henry and Stephens (1977) describe two major responses of the
individual to a perceived stimulus, mediated by the limbic system (see
Figure 4). The threat to control leads to a fight-flight response
mediated by the amygdala. In contrast a sense of loss of control, and

failure to meet expectations, leads to depression followed by
conservation-withdrawal mediated by the hippocampus-septum. The
physiological-endocrine consequences of these two response patterns
differ, as shown in Figure 5 (Henry, 1987). Carroll's discoveries of
elevated plasma cortisol and an abnormal dexamethasone suppression test in
patients with primary depression, lends support to this hypothesis
(Carroll, 1976).

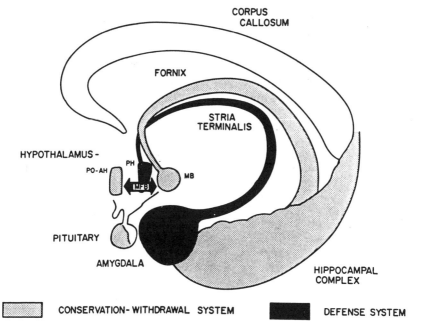

CONSERVATION-WITHDRAWAL SYSTEM   DEFENSE SYSTEM

FIGURE 4: This highly schematic diagram shows the relation of two
important temporal lobe structures to the hypothalamus. It
depicts the connections of the hippocampus and contrasts them
with those of the amygdala. (PO-AH = Preoptic Anterior
Hypothalamic Region, PH = Posterior Hypothalamus, MFB = Medial
Forebrain Bundle, MB = Mammillary Body). From Henry, J.P. and
Stephens, P.M. (1977). Stress, Health and the Social
Environment - A Sociobiological Approach to Medicine. New
York: Springer-Verlag. With Permission.

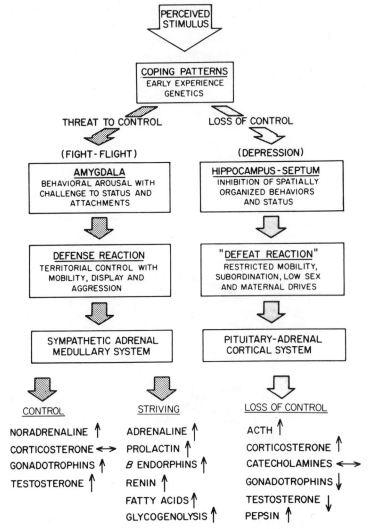

FIGURE 5: The defense response and the sympatho-adrenal system are activated when the organism is challenged and in control of the environment. By contrast, loss of territorial control and failure to meet expectations involves the adrenal cortical system as the defeat reaction takes over. From Henry, J.P. (1987). Psychological factors and coronary heart disease. Holistic Medicine. 2, 119-132. With Permission.

These response patterns are of particular relevance when one considers the varying behavioural changes in individuals with dementia and other brain diseases. Certainly any conditions which affect cognition and intellectual functioning can lead to a realistic perception of a serious threat to one's sense of control or to a feeling of loss of control over one's environment. Whether individuals with Alzheimer's disease for example, become hostile and belligerent, as opposed to withdrawn and depressed, might relate to a combination of factors including premorbid personality, previous levels of self-esteem, response of family and/or staff and also perhaps to specific cell loss occurring in localized areas of the limbic system, with associated behavioural consequences.

THE EFFECTS OF AGING ON THE BRAIN

It has been calculated that the human cerebral cortex contains 16.5 thousand million nerve cells, of which about 100,000 are believed to die off every day (Platt, 1986). In an 80 year life span the mean loss of neurons in the brain therefore would amount to about 3% of the neurons present at birth. However, it has been demonstrated that in certain parts of the brain, such as the thalamus, up to 18% of cells are lost during normal aging (Platt, 1986). Furthermore, the white matter shrinks in old age about twice as much as the gray matter. Thus, with regard to loss of brain weight in the elderly, the major part of the loss of substance affects the white conduction pathways, rather than the gray matter. Neuropathological changes similar to those seen in Alzheimer's disease are found in the elderly on post-mortem examination. These changes are, however, much less widespread. This might suggest that Alzheimer's disease represents an acceleration of the aging process, but this is an unproven theory (Strub and Black, 1981). Reports of changes in brain metabolism associated with aging *per se* are somewhat difficult to interpret, because it is difficult to control for age-related neuropathology. However, a significant decline in cerebral energy metabolism with age has been shown in many, but not all studies.

Aging appears to be associated with diminished concentrations of dopamine, norepinephrine and serotonin within the brain as well as a decrease in cholineacetyltransferase, tyrosine hydroxylase and dopamine decarboxylase. Concentrations of monoamine oxidase increase, which may lead to greater vulnerability to depression in the elderly.

There is much controversy regarding the effect of aging on specific intellectual functions. Certain intellectual functions may actually improve rather than decline with age. Activities which demand associative mental functioning, such as relating new information to previously accumulated knowledge, fall into this category, including general knowledge, practical judgement and dexterity with vocabulary and language. Other abilities, such as concentration, mental agility and some right hemisphere functions, appear to be less age resistant. Several studies have demonstrated that scores on the verbal subtests of the Wechsler Adult Intelligence Scale (WAIS) remained relatively stable with age, whereas scores on the performance subtests declined (Wechsler, 1958; Eisdorfer, Busse and Cohen, 1959). This pattern of preservation of verbal abilities, with decline in non-verbal abilities, has been referred to as the "classical aging pattern" (Hochanadel and Kaplan, 1984).

PSYCHIATRIC DISEASE IN THE ELDERLY

In considering neuropsychiatric problems in the elderly, it is important to reflect briefly on psychiatric illness in the aging population. The elderly are not immune from any of the psychiatric disorders which afflict younger adults. Despite popular belief that depression is rampant in the elderly, evidence suggests that the point prevalence rate for major depression is about 2% at age 65 years and above (Angst, 1986). For minor and secondary depressive disorders in this age group, it is somewhere between 5 and 15% (Angst, 1986). In other words, there is no evidence that major depressive disorders increase with age. In fact, the rates may be somewhat lower in old age than during the mid-life. In contrast, the evidence suggests that suicide rates increase almost linearly with age.

It is clear that a number of psychological and social factors may influence the development of depression in the elderly. Old age is a time of increasing loss and, potentially, of declining self-esteem, generated in part by the societal attitude towards the elderly, which, particularly in western countries, may result in ageism. Apart from the problems of diagnosing depression in the medically ill, it may be hard to differentiate mild dysphoria or demoralization from significant clinical depression in the elderly. There is evidence that late life depressions are qualitatively different from depression earlier in life. For example, the elderly seem to experience guilt-ridden depression less frequently than younger individuals, while delusional depression occurs more often. Masked depression (i.e. depression without sadness or dysphoria) and somatic complaints appear to be more frequent in the elderly.

Mania in the elderly appears to be relatively rare. In elderly bipolar patients whose first manic attack occurred at age 60 or over, particularly among men, there appears to be a preponderance of cerebral organic disorders (Shulman and Post, 1980). There is evidence that a variety of medical diseases and drugs can cause secondary mania (Krauthammer and Klerman, 1978). A review of reported cases of mania secondary to localized brain pathology revealed that most focal lesions were associated with disorders of the diencephalic region of the brain and that the majority of lateralized lesions were in the right hemisphere (Cummings and Mendez, 1984).

Psychotic disorders in the elderly can occur in a variety of disorders including paranoid disorders, schizophrenia and organic disorders. Paranoid symptomatology in general is a major presenting complaint among elderly psychiatric patients (Pfeiffer, 1977). Psychosis is also associated with medical disorders where the potentially complicating overlap with delirium may create diagnostic difficulties. Cummings (1988) has reviewed the literature regarding the association between delusional disorders and medical/organic illness. Paraphrenia is a particular form of paranoid, psychotic disorder occurring for the first time later in life. This usually involves the development of a fixed, relatively encapsulated, paranoid, delusional belief and most frequently occurs in those living alone and having sensory, particularly hearing, loss. Paraphrenia is difficult to treat because patients frequently refuse anti-psychotic treatment.

CLASSIFICATION OF NEUROPSYCHIATRIC SYNDROMES

The coining of the terms "dementia" and "delirium" has been attributed to the Roman, Celsus, in his work De Medicina (1st century A.D.) (Lipowski, 1981). The term dementia was used to refer both to a syndrome of psychological delapadation (in a clinical sense) and to the state of civil and legal incapacity (a forensic meaning) (Berrios, 1987). By the late 18th century, dementia was a common term but was used in a rather nonspecific sense. The term senile dementia was used by Esquirol in the 19th century (Torack, 1983). He described 3 forms of dementia - acute, chronic and senile.

With advances in neuropathology at the turn of the century, there were considerable changes in the concept of dementia. Alzheimer and Pick described clinical disorders characterized by memory and behavioural disturbance and linked these changes to neuropathological findings. The term Alzheimer's Disease was originally used with reference to middle-aged patients, and was also termed pre-senile dementia. Subsequently, as it became recognized that the neuropathology of older patients with dementia was identical to younger patients, the term "senile dementia of the Alzheimer's type" evolved.

The diagnostic and statistical manual of mental disorders of the American Psychiatric Association was revised in 1980 with the publication of DSM-III, and included major innovations in the diagnosis of organic mental disorders. Organic brain syndromes had been defined in DSM-II as those mental disorders which were caused by or were associated with impairment of brain tissue function. They were stated to be characterized by the basic organic brain syndrome, whose essential features included impairment of orientation, all intellectual functions, memory and judgement and lability or shallowness of affect. The DSM-III task force felt that these descriptions were restrictive and made it impossible to include many psychopathological manifestations of cerebral disorders.

The latest revision of the DSM-III, entitled DSM-III-R was published in 1987 (American Psychiatric Association, 1987). In DSM-III-R a distinction is made between organic mental syndromes and organic mental disorders. The term organic mental *syndrome* is used to refer to a constellation of psychological or behavioural signs and symptoms, without reference to etiology. Organic mental *disorder* designates a particular organic mental syndrome in which the etiology is known or presumed. The essential feature of all disorders is a psychological or behavioural abnormality associated with transient or permanent dysfunction of the brain. The organic factor responsible for an organic mental disorder may be a primary disease of the brain or a systemic illness that secondarily affects the brain. Intoxication or withdrawal from a psychoactive substance can also be responsible for an organic mental disorder. The diagnosis of an organic mental disorder is made by recognizing the presence of one of the organic mental syndromes, and by demonstrating by means of the history, physical examination or laboratory tests, the presence of a specific organic factor (or factors) judged to be etiologically related to the abnormal mental state.

The organic mental syndromes can be grouped into six categories:
1.   Delirium and dementia, in which cognitive impairment is relatively global.
2.   Amnestic syndrome and organic hallucinosis, in which relatively selective areas of cognition are impaired.
3.   Organic delusional syndrome, organic mood syndrome and organic anxiety syndrome, which have features resembling schizophrenic, mood and anxiety disorders.
4.   Organic personality syndrome in which the personality is affected.
5.   Intoxication and withdrawal of a psychoactive substance.
6.   Organic mental syndrome not otherwise specified, which is a residual category.

The diagnostic criteria for delirium and dementia are delineated in Tables 1 and 2. The essential features of delirium include reduced ability to maintain attention to external stimuli and to appropriately shift attention to new external stimuli, and disorganized thinking. The syndrome may also involve a reduced level of consciousness, sensory

TABLE 1: DIAGNOSTIC CRITERIA FOR DELIRIUM. Reprinted with Permission From the Diagnostic and Statistical Manual of Mental Disorders. Third Edition. Revised. Copyright 1987. American Psychiatric Association.

A. Reduced ability to maintain attention to external stimuli (e.g., questions must be repeated because attention wanders) and to appropriately shift attention to new external stimuli (e.g., perseverates answer to a previous question).

B. Disorganized thinking, as indicated by rambling, irrelevant, or incoherent speech.

C. At least two of the following:
    (1) reduced level of consciousness, e.g., difficulty keeping awake during examination

    (2) perceptual disturbances: misinterpretations, illusions, or hallucinations

    (3) disturbance of sleep-wake cycle with insomnia or daytime sleepiness

    (4) increased or decreased psychomotor activity

    (5) disorientation to time, place or person

    (6) memory impairment, e.g., inability to learn new material, such as the names of several unrelated objects after five minutes, or to remember past events, such as history of current episode of illness

D. Clinical features develop over a short period of time (usually hours to days) and tend to fluctuate over the course of a day.

E. Either (1) or (2):

    (1) evidence from the history, physical examination, or laboratory tests of a specific organic factor (or factors) judged to be etiologically related to the disturbance

    (2) in the absence of such evidence, an etiologic organic factor can be presumed if the disturbance cannot be accounted for by any nonorganic mental disorder, e.g., Manic Episode accounting for agitation and sleep disturbance

TABLE 2:   DIAGNOSTIC CRITERIA FOR DEMENTIA. Reprinted
with Permission from the Diagnostic and Statistical
Manual of Mental Disorders. Third Edition. Revised.
Copyright 1987. American Psychiatric Association.

A.   Demonstrable evidence of impairment in short and long-term
memory. Impairment in short-term memory (inability to learn
new information) may be indicated by inability to remember three
objects after five minutes. Long-term memory impairment
(inability to remember information that was known in the past)
may be indicated by inability to remember past personal
information (e.g., past Presidents, well-known dates).

B.   At least one of the following:

(1)   impairment in abstract thinking, as indicated by inability to
find similarities and differences between related words,
difficulty in defining words and concepts, and other similar
tasks

(2)   impaired judgment, as indicated by inability to make
reasonable plans to deal with interpersonal, family, and
job-related problems and issues

(3)   other disturbances of higher cortical function, such as
aphasia (disorder of language), apraxia (inability to carry
out motor activities despite intact comprehension and motor
function), and "constructional difficulty" (e.g., inability
to copy three-dimensional figures, assemble blocks, or
arrange sticks in specific designs)

(4)   personality change, i.e., alteration or accentuation of
premorbid traits

C.   The disturbance in A and B significantly interferes with work or
usual social activities or relationships with others.

D.   Not occurring exclusively during the course of Delirium.

E.   Either (1) or (2):

(1)   there is evidence from the history, physical examination, or
laboratory tests of a specific organic factor (or factors)
judged to be etiologically related to the disturbance

(2)   in the absence of such evidence, an etiologic organic factor
can be presumed if the disturbance cannot be accounted for by
any nonorganic mental disorder, e.g., Major Depression
accounting for cognitive impairment

misperceptions, disturbances of the sleep-wake cycle and level of psychomotor activity, disorientation to time, place, or person, and memory impairment. The essential feature of dementia is impairment in memory, both short and long term, associated with impairment in abstract thinking, impaired judgement, other disturbances of higher cortical function, or personality change. The disturbance is severe enough to interfere significantly with work or usual social activities or relationships with others.

In the other organic mental syndromes the areas of dysfunction are more discrete. Memory is the major dysfunction in the amnestic syndrome. Organic delusional syndrome is characterized by prominent delusions, and organic hallucinosis by persistant or recurrent hallucinations. In organic mood syndrome the phenomenology is similar to that of a manic or major depressive episode. This syndrome can be subdivided into either manic, depressed or mixed categories. In organic anxiety syndrome panic attacks or generalized anxiety occur. In organic personality syndrome there must be a persistant personality disturbance characterized by at least one of the following: affective instability; recurrent outbursts of aggression or rage; markedly impaired social judgement; marked apathy and indifference; suspiciousness or paranoid ideation. A subcategory in the case of outbursts of aggression or rage has been categorized as "explosive type". In each of the above syndromes there must be evidence of a specific organic factor (or factors) judged to be etiologically related to the disturbance.

Etiology of Organic Mental Disorders

The most common causes of delirium are metabolic disorders, systemic infections, hepatic or renal disease, post-operative states and psycho-active substance intoxication or withdrawal. The most common cause of dementia is senile dementia of the Alzheimer type, followed by multi-infarct dementia. There are also a variety of potentially reversible conditions including central nervous system infections, brain trauma eg. subdural hematoma, toxic metabolic disturbances, and normal pressure hydrocephalus. Dementia may also occur secondary to a number of neurologic diseases such as Huntington's chorea, multiple sclerosis, Parkinson's disease or progessive supranuclear palsy.

Amnestic syndrome may result from bilateral damage to certain diencephalic and medial temporal structures. The most common form of the syndrome is associated with chronic alcohol abuse and vitamin deficiency. Other causes include head trauma, hypoxia, herpes simplex encephalitis and infarction in the territories of the posterior cerebral arteries.

The most common causes of organic delusional syndrome include psycho-active substances such as amphetamines and hallucinogens, temporal lobe epilepsy, and Huntington's chorea. There may be a specific relationship between right hemisphere cerebral lesions and this syndrome. In the elderly, the most common cause of organic hallucinosis is probably sensory deprivation, which can occur with blindness or deafness. Many elderly patients with a visual disturbance such as cataracts develop extremely vivid and often frightening visual hallucinations (Rosenbaum, Harati, Rolak, and Freedman, 1987). Alcohol and hallucinogens are also common causes of this syndrome.

Organic mood syndrome may be caused by neurological diseases such as stroke, carcinoma, especially of the pancreas, viral illnesses, endocrine disorders, particularly thyroid and adrenal dysfunction, and a variety of toxic or metabolic factors, including certain medications such as anti-hypertensives. Organic anxiety syndrome may be caused by endocrine disorders particularly hyperthyroidism, pheochromocytoma, hypoglycemia and hypercortisolism. Other causes include intoxication from stimulants such as caffeine, cocaine and amphetamines, or withdrawal from substances such as alcohol and sedatives. Common etiologies of organic personality syndrome include frontal lobe damage and temporal lobe epilepsy.

Lipowski (1984), in discussing the new approach of the DSM-III to organic mental disorders, noted that the essential feature of organic mental disorders is no longer cognitive or intellectual impairment but "the psychological or behavioural abnormality associated with transient or permanent dysfuntion of the brain". The concept of organic disorders has been expanded and liberalized. No longer is the concept of organicity synonymous with the presence of cognitive impairment. The previous delineation of acute and chronic syndromes has been abandoned because it forces a clinician to classify a patient's organic brain syndrome as either reversible or not, on the basis of only a cross-sectional assessment. Lipowski (1984) pointed out that it is a fallacy to conceive of reversibility of cognitive impairment as an all-or-none phenomenon. Instead, it should be viewed as a spectrum ranging from full restoration, through varying degrees of partial resolution, to progressive and irreversible deterioration.

Although this new classification system appears to be a major advance in the field there have been a number of criticisms levelled against it. The new approach has been accused of blurring the traditional distinction between organic and functional psychopathology. It has been suggested that the new classification is over-inclusive and overly complex, that it might hinder case finding for epidemiological studies, that it imposes premature closure on the issue of cause and leaves too much to the clinician's judgement (Spitzer, Williams and Skodol, 1983). Indeed, this is the only section of the DSM-III in which the clinician is asked to make an etiological diagnosis.

DIAGNOSTIC PROBLEMS

One of the practical difficulties of diagnosis is the tendency for patients with neuropsychiatric disorders to have atypical or mixed symptoms that do not easily fit into the standard classification systems. The diagnosis of depression is, of course, of the utmost importance and no clinician wants to miss an eminently treatable condition. The diagnosis of depression and other psychiatric disorders in patients with brain disease can be fraught with difficulties (Ross and Rush, 1981). The affect itself can be one of the most misleading aspects of the mental state examination. Frequently a psychiatrist may be consulted because a patient has labile depressive affect, that is, crying very easily. The regulation of affect, and the prosody of speech, may be altered by primary brain disease. Prosody is the affective and inflectional colouring of speech, including syllable and word stress, rhythm, cadence and pitch. These aspects, as well as gesture and mimicry, provide the emotional element to speech.

Dysprosody distorts the patient's ability to communicate emotional states. Prosody can be disturbed by right hemisphere lesions and by disorders of the basal ganglia, cerebellum and brain stem. This may lead to a flat, monotonous voice and can lead to either an under or over-estimation of the severity of an emotional disorder such as depression. The flat monotonous voice may be mistaken for depression or conversely, the examiner may be unconvinced of depression when the patient is genuinely feeling sad and melancholic.

In the presence of dysprosody, it is clearly important to maximize communication with a patient, especially if cognitive impairment, sensory deficits or aphasia are present (Conn, 1986). It may be important to remove interfering noise, and to make hearing aids, letterboards and interpreters available. It is important to obtain corroborative history from family and professional staff and the examiner should try to get a picture of the patient's premorbid personality and functioning. A past psychiatric history, especially of depression and of family history, should be obtained.

A number of common conditions may cause diagnostic confusion. For example, the patient with Parkinsonism and masked facies may be mistakenly thought of as depressed. An agitated and disinhibited patient with frontal lobe damage, may be thought of as being manic. Patients with aphasia, particularly fluent aphasia, may appear to have a thought disorder. Pseudobulbar affect (loss of control of emotions as a result of brain disease) may be confused with depression, although some authors believe that this may actually indicate an underlying depressive disorder (Ross and Rush, 1981).

PSYCHIATRIC CONSEQUENCES OF SPECIFIC NEUROLOGICAL DISEASES

Stroke

As early as 1924, Bleuler described melancholic moods following stroke. There has been growing interest in the relationship between mood disorder and stroke, and a considerable amount of research into this relationship, particularly in the last decade, has been spearheaded by Robert Robinson. Several studies have tried to determine whether depression following stroke was a specific complication of that disorder. Robins (1976) did not find that stroke patients were any more depressed than other disabled subjects, however Folstein, Maiberger and McHugh (1977) found that stroke patients were more depressed than orthopedic patients with similar degrees of disability (45% vs. 10%). Patients with right hemisphere stroke seemed particularly vulnerable and displayed a syndrome of irritability, loss of interest and difficulty in concentration, in addition to depression of mood. Some patients with right hemisphere lesions also have an indifferent apathetic mental state associated with inappropriate cheerfulness (Robinson, Kubos, Starr, Rao and Price, 1983).

Several studies by Robinson and his group have led to the conclusion that patients with left hemisphere strokes are more vulnerable to depressive syndromes, particularly if the lesion is close to the frontal pole (Robinson, Kubos, Starr, Rao and Price, 1983; Robinson, Lipsey, Kolla-Wilson, Bolduc, Pearlson, Rao and Price, 1985). However, most studies have failed to show a consistent association between side of lesion and the presence of depression (House, 1987). In one study (Robinson, Starr, Kubos and Price, 1983) 26% of a group of 103 stroke patients had the symptoms of major depression and another 20% had symptoms of minor (dysthymic) depression. At subsequent examinations six months later, 34% had symptoms of major depression, 26% had minor depression and only 40% remained non-depressed (Robinson, Starr and Price, 1984). Follow-up studies suggest that the high risk period for post-stroke depression lasts approximately two years.

Robinson also examined the relationship between depression and other factors. He found that 50%, or more, of the variance in depression can be explained by lesion location, whereas only 15% of the variance can be explained by severity of intellectual impairment, severity of physical impairment, quality of available social supports or age. Robinson, using a model of stroke in the rat, interestingly demonstrated that a small localized lesion of the cortex will produce wide-spread depletions of norepinephrine *throughout* the brain (Robinson, 1979). In addition, he found, surprisingly, that the neurochemical response may be lateralized. These findings suggest that depletion of biogenic amines, particularly following injury to anterior regions of the brain, may contribute to the etiology of post-stroke depression.

The results of two studies suggest that anti-depressants may have an important role in the treatment of depression following stroke. Lipsey, Robinson, Pearlson, Rao and Price (1984) found that nortriptyline was significantly more effective than placebo. Reding, Orto and Winter (1986) discovered that only patients with abnormal dexamethasone suppression tests improved significantly more with trazodone than with placebo and these patients also showed greater improvement in activity of daily living scores. Murray, Shea and Conn (1986) suggest that ECT can also be effective and relatively safe in the treatment of depressed patients with a history of stroke.

Much of the work in this area has focused on depression following stroke. There have been few studies of anxiety following stroke. It is clear, however, that many patients are extremely fearful following a stroke, with a variety of realistic fears, including the fear of having another stroke or of dying, or of becoming permanently paralysed, handicapped or totally dependent. Mesulam (1979) noted that patients who have had strokes without hemiplegia may initially present with behavioural abnormalities or deficits in language and memory alone. He described, for example, the acute onset of incoherent language and bizarre behaviour following a left temporo-parietal infarction, the acute onset of agitated delirium following medial occipito-temporal infarction, and the acute onset of confusion without agitation or acute derangements of insight, judgement and comportment following a right hemisphere infarction. A syndrome of delayed psychosis after right temporo-parietal stroke or trauma has been described (Levine and Finklestein 1982). The patients developed hallucinations and in some cases delusions and severe agitation. Interestingly, seven out of eight patients had clinical seizures in close temporal relationship to the psychosis.

From a clinical viewpoint, it is important to note that the sudden development of a stroke can be a devastating and terrifying experience, particularly if the individual is aware of the developing loss of function. Eric Hodgins in his book "Episode: Report on the Accident inside my Skull" described vividly, his experiences following a stroke, in which he became aphasic (Hodgins, 1964). "To my shock and incredulity, I could not speak. That is, I could utter nothing intelligible. All that would come from my lips was the sound ab, which I repeated again and again and again."

Case No.1. An 82-year-old man with a history of ischemic heart disease and myocardial infarctions was referred to the psychiatric team one week after a left hemisphere stroke, because of severe depression and loss of appetite. He had been seen previously by the psychiatric consultation service because of a period of depression during an episode of congestive heart failure. At that time his depression had lifted quickly as his medical condition improved. On the second occasion, nursing staff described him as difficult to look after, and noted that he was demanding and hostile. He voiced depressive thoughts including the fact that he no longer wanted to live. His wife had had Alzheimer's Disease for 5 years and was in a nursing home. He had two children and evidently had a difficult relationship with one of them.

He presented as an angry, impatient and hostile man, who repeated over and over "get me out of here". He was extremely depressed, hopeless and had given up. He said that he had nothing left to live for and asked the psychiatrist to give him poison. He said that it would be better if his right arm was cut off, as it was now useless. He felt that he was useless and had nothing left to contribute. He would discuss nothing else. He refused to answer questions with regard to specific cognitive function. Aphasia did not appear to be a significant problem.

Recommendations included treatment with nortriptyline (up to 30 mg/day) and the use of a sitter to help support and encourage him. His condition continued to deteriorate and his depression did not respond to the anti-depressant. His statements included "Leave me alone. I have lived enough. I don't have anything to live for. Give me poison." and "Leave me to die. I'm going to kill myself. I hope your children will suffer the way that I do. Why are you doing this to me?" and "Leave me alone. Don't treat me like an animal. Kill me instead. No, go away." and "What crime did I do? I didn't kill anybody. Why are you punishing me? How long can a person take this?"

The team decided to treat his condition vigorously. Intravenous fluids were administered and subsequently a nasogastric tube was inserted for feeding. He spent much of his time shutting out the world with his eyes closed. Four weeks after his stroke, he had a cardiac arrest and died.

This case raised a number of anguishing ethical, moral and philosophical questions for the treatment team. It was apparent soon after his stroke that the patient had given up. (It is the author's experience that the vast majority of patients who have totally and genuinely "given-up", do not respond to anti-depressant treatment). He certainly appeared to have a classical depression but the standard interventions for the treatment of depression had no effect. He clearly stated that he wanted to die. Should the treatment team have been as aggressive as they were? Should more aggressive measures have been taken? Did he "die with dignity"?

Case No.2. A 64-year-old, right-handed, single female presented to the Emergency department following an episode of loss of speech, accompanied by dizziness and generalized weakness. Her past medical history included mild polio at age 34, a recent left-sided Bell's palsy and hypertension. Neurological findings included a slight, left-sided facial droop, a partial left ptosis and a slight left-sided hemiparesis, all of which were long-standing. Her speech was slow, hesitant and slightly garbled. Soon after admission, she developed a dense, right, homonomous hemianopia and a bilateral internuclear ophthalmoplegia.

Over the next few days her speech slowly improved, although she remained dysarthric. Subsequently, she became increasingly talkative and her mood was somewhat labile. Her neurologist questioned the possibility of hypomania. A CT scan demonstrated a small area of low density in the left frontal corona, consistent with an old infarction and moderate cerebral atrophy. She was discharged, but 8 days later was brought to the Emergency because of episodes of immobility. She was re-admitted and developed a syndrome of akinesia, mutism and unresponsiveness suggestive of a depressive stupor. CT scan revealed a sub-acute, left occipital infarct.

Two days after admission she became more alert and spoke to staff. She denied feeling depressed but appeared sad and said she was disgusted with herself because she was taking so long to recover from the stroke. Her course was characterized by periods of akinesia and mutism. She was treated with maprotiline and gradually seemed more alert. On the 8th day after beginning this medication she became active, talkative and appeared euthymic. She remained more alert but was still periodically mute.

She was discharged home but two weeks later was readmitted, akinetic and unresponsive. A brief trial of methylphenidate did not alter her condition. Several sodium amytal interviews produced equivocal results. Two weeks after admission she became increasingly agitated

with unintelligible speech, reminiscent of "talking in tongues". She
appeared to be fearful and visually hallucinating. Oral intake
remained minimal. The differential diagnosis included psychotic
depression and delirium. Metabolic and toxic etiologies were ruled
out. She was treated with haloperidol for sedation, in low dosage.
This reduced her agitation but she remained withdrawn and required
nasogastric tube feedings.

Because of the life-threatening nature of this syndrome, the lack of
the response to pharmacological treatment and evidence suggesting an
atypical affective disorder, she was treated with a course of ECT.
She received seven unilateral treatments over a two week period.
After the fifth treatment there was a dramatic change. She started to
talk, was completely appropriate and rational and started to eat a
full diet. She was discharged home seven weeks after admission.

This case points to the difficulty of trying to classify a patient
with a neuropsychiatric syndrome of this nature using conventional
psychiatric diagnoses. Although she had many features of depression
this would clearly represent an atypical form of affective disorder.
This patient, on clinical examination, had features of a brain stem
lesion, which may have disrupted certain ascending pathways and
contributed to her state of stupor. The fact that the patient
appeared to respond to ECT, does not confirm the diagnosis of an
affective disorder, although it does suggest that her disorder may
have been related to a neurotransmitter disturbance.

Parkinson's Disease

The most common form of Parkinson's disease is idiopathic
parkinsonism, also termed paralysis agitans. The major features are
tremor, muscular rigidity, hypokinesis and abnormal posture. The etiology
is thought to be a degeneration of pigmented cells in the brain stem,
particularly in the substantia nigra. Known etiologies of parkinsonism
include certain medications (neuroleptics, methyl-dopa and reserpine),
encephalitis and arteriosclerosis. Studies suggest that more than 80% of
cases are idiopathic in origin (Hoehn & Yahr, 1967). The condition is
usually progressive. In this study, 25% of patients were severely
disabled or dead within five years of onset and two-thirds within ten
years.

Depression is known to be frequently associated with Parkinson's
disease. However, the results of studies of frequency vary considerably,
with some suggesting that up to 70% of sufferers are depressed. Studies
have found that depressed patients with Parkinson's disease have lower
levels of 5-hydroxyindoleacetic acid in their cerebral spinal fluid than

do non-depressed Parkinsonians (Mayeux, Stern, Cote, and Williams, 1984). Fibiger (1984) proposed that degeneration of mesolimbic and mesocortical dopamine projections may account for the anhedonia and depression. Most studies suggest that the degree of physical disability, the age of the patient and the duration of the disease, do not seem to correlate with the severity of depression (Horn, 1974; Celesia and Wanamaker, 1972). In a recent study comparing elderly patients with Parkinson's disease and with arthritis, Gotham, Brown, and Marsden, (1986) found that, although the patients with Parkinson's disease showed significantly higher levels of depression compared to normal controls, they did not differ from those patients with arthritis. Both groups had depression characterized by pessimism, hopelessness, and decreased motivation and drive. However, the negative affects of guilt, self-blame and worthlessness were absent in both patient groups. In this study, the pattern of depression *was* significantly associated with the severity of illness and functional disability, although these factors accounted for only a modest proportion of the variability in test scores.

New studies are critically examining the qualitative aspects of depression in patients with Parkinsonism. (Taylor, Saint-Cyr, Lang and Kenny, 1986). Diagnosis can be difficult because the masked facies and slowed movement of these patients may confound the assessment of affect and mood. Of particular importance is the fact that the depression has been found to improve with antidepressants and ECT. There has even been some suggestion that ECT may also help the motor symptoms of Parkinson's disease. Recent studies suggest that deprenyl, a selective monoamine-oxidase-B inhibitor might be helpful in the treatment of Parkinson's disease by slowing down the catabolism of dopamine and possibly allowing a decrease in the dosage of levodopa required to control the symptoms of the disease (Ruggieri, Stocchi, Denaro, Baronti and Agnoli, 1986).

Studies suggest that schizophrenia-like psychosis in association with Parkinson's disease is rare (Davison and Bagley, 1969). Celesia and Wanamaker (1972) found acute psychotic symptoms in 12% of 153 patients. These symptoms were generally attributable to medications used to treat the primary disease and occurred most frequently in patients who were cognitively impaired. In another study Klawans, Moskovitz, Nausieda and Weiner (1979) found that 48% of patients using levodopa developed at least one psychiatric symptom over the course of one year. Vivid dreams were very common and were associated with visual hallucinations in some patients. Paranoid delusion occurred in 9% of patients. Hypersexuality, although it is an often described symptom, actually occurs in less than 1% of patients. The possibility that the psychosis of chronic levodopa therapy may be caused by dopaminergic kindling has been suggested (Moskovitz, Moses and Klawans, 1978). Another hypothesis is that psychotic symptoms are triggered by the action of dopamine as a false transmitter at serotonergic receptors (Birkmayer & Riederer 1975).

Case No.3. A 78-year-old widower, a retired accountant and nursing home resident, with a six year history of Parkinson's disease, was referred to psychiatry because of inappropriate sexual comments to the staff. He subsequently described his belief that the night staff were engaged in parties on the unit, late at night. He believed that they had a belly-dancer and was dismayed that he was excluded from these activities. He also described a long history of impotence. For a period of time he was quite disturbed by these thoughts. The most rational approach to the treatment of delusions or hallucinations in patients receiving anti-parkinsonian medication is a gradual and careful reduction in the dosage of this medication. However, in this case it was felt that his already marginal mobility would be severely compromised by such a step. A trial of a low dose neuroleptic (thioridazine 10 mg bid) exacerbated his Parkinsonian symptoms and was therefore discontinued. He subsequently became less concerned about these delusional thoughts. Two years later he developed paranoid thoughts that family members had been stealing his clothes. In spite of this he continued to attend programs and social events. Neuroleptics were not recommended. Decisions with regard to the treatment of psychosis in Parkinson's patients must be carefully considered. There is some evidence that new neuroleptic drugs with more specific dopamine blocking activity do not cause a worsening of motor symptoms. These agents are not in general use because of other side effects, however, they hopefully herald an era of new medications whose specific actions will reduce the potentially negative effects in this patient population.

Case No.4. A 76-year-old married woman of Russian origin was admitted to hospital with a four year history of progressive Parkinson's disease. She was referred because of agitation, belligerence, and threats that she would jump out of the window. She had been married for 43 years and the couple seemed very devoted to each other. They had no children. One year earlier a psychologist had noted only mild signs of cognitive impairment. There had also been evidence of depression with low mood, sleep disturbance, weight gain, decreased energy, loss of concentration and fears of being a cripple. She related that she had lost her vitality, physical beauty and interest in self-care. She had been admitted to a Geriatric Psychiatric Day Hospital and treated briefly with antidepressants. However, her Parkinsonian condition deteriorated, leading to admission to a rehabilitation floor. Medications included levodopa/carbidopa 100/25, 6 tablets per day. On admission she was wheelchair bound, disoriented, restless and agitated. She whispered answers and frequently looked away, as if distracted, although she denied hallucinations. She would initially answer questions in English, but repeatedly switched to Russian. Her translator said that she made some sense but that her ideas were disconnected. She seemed fearful and wanted desperately to go home. She was thought to be severely demented and applications were made for nursing homes.

When the patient's levodopa/carbidopa was reduced to 4 tablets a day there was a remarkable change in her condition. She became less agitated, more oriented, and increasingly cooperative in her rehabilitation, to the point of improved mobilization. After six weeks in hospital she was discharged home. She appeared to have been suffering from a delirium secondary to excessive levodopa. It is of critical importance to rule out iatrogenesis in patients with Parkinson's disease (or other neurological diseases) who display psychiatric symptoms.

The Dementias

The DSM-III-R definition of dementia, as described above, remains a topic of considerable debate. Alexander and Geschwind (1984) suggest that the term dementia does not have a sharp boundary, that it refers to a loosely similar group of disabilities, in which there is deterioration in one or more behavioural functions, that leads to an inability to carry out reasonably independent activity.

Studies suggest that about 50% of patients referred to neurologists for evaluation of dementia will show evidence of a degenerative brain disease, most commonly Alzheimer's Disease. The next three diagnoses in order of frequency are: multi-infarct dementia, depressive pseudodementia and the effects of alcohol (Marsden and Harrison, 1972; Freemon, 1976). Other important causes of dementia in the elderly include normal pressure hydrocephalus (potentially treatable with a ventricular shunt), and Pick's disease. Alzheimer's Disease is the most common cause of dementia and is generally a relentlessly progressive condition. It is more frequent in women than in men. Pathological changes include senile plaques, neurofibrillary tangles and granulovacuolar degeneration. Neuronal loss is most marked in the hippocampus, neocortical association areas, medial amygdala and nucleus basalis of Meynert. From a neuropsychiatric standpoint, one of the most challenging and intriguing issues regarding the patient with dementia, is the differentiation from and the co-existence of depression.

The task of differentiating depression from dementia is of critical importance and yet on occasion, exceedingly difficult. Depression and dementia can, of course, coexist. Depression seems to occur frequently in

the course of pre-senile dementia (Sim and Sussman, 1962). In a study of
88 cognitively impaired elderly outpatients, depression occurred in 17
patients (Reifler, Larson and Hanley, 1982). Depression was most frequent
in patients with mild dementia. Another study, which excluded patients
with a history of depression or with current evidence of depression, found
no evidence that the remaining patients developed significant degrees of
depression over a twelve month period (Knesevish, Martin, Berg and
Danziger, 1983).

The incidence of depression in different forms of dementia remains
uncertain. A clinician must be aware of the possiblity that cognitive
impairment, secondary to depression, may mimic dementia, leading to the so
called syndrome of pseudodementia. In this situation the term dementia
syndrome of depression is also applied. Madden described 10% of 300
patients, aged 45 and older in a psychiatric unit who had "pseudodementia"
(Madden, Luhan, Kaplan, and Manfredi, 1952). The term "pseudodementia"
can only be applied in retrospect, i.e. following recovery or improvement.

Pseudodementia is not limited to patients with affective disorders;
other psychiatric diagnoses such as hysteria are also considered to cause
the syndrome (Kiloh, 1961). In one retrospective study of 35 patients
with the diagnosis of pre-senile dementia, on long term follow-up 20 did
not develop degenerative dementia (Nott and Fleminger, 1975). Three of
the patients were depressed and others had different psychiatric diagnoses
such as anxiety, hysteria and paranoid disorders. A 5 to 15 year follow-
up of 52 patients with a diagnosis of pre-senile dementia revealed that
31% of the group had been misdiagnosed (Ron, Toone, Garralda and Lishman,
1979). In another study of 106 patients referred to a neurological
hospital with the diagnosis of dementia, 14% had no evidence of cognitive
impairment on psychological testing, and slightly more than half of these
patients had evidence of depression (Marsden and Harrison, 1972).

Wells (1979) listed a series of clinical findings that might be
helpful in distinguishing pseudodementia from dementia. These features of
pseudodementia included a distinct date of onset, rapid progression,
previous psychiatric history and an intense awareness by family of the
patient's impairment. Patients with pseudodementia were more likely to
complain about their intellectual decline and to demonstrate poor effort
and inconsistency in psychological testing. Affective symptoms are more
evident, with early loss of social skills and absence of nocturnal
exacerbation of symptoms ("sundowning"). Patients are more likely to
respond with "I don't know" answers, and display equally impaired recent
and remote memory. However, it has been shown that no clinical finding is
pathagnomonic of either of the two conditions (McAllister and Price,
1982). A past history of depression or a positive family history of
depression should raise the clinician's level of suspicion. It has been

suggested that even if the patient recovers, subsequent development of dementia is not uncommon (Kral, 1983).

Case No.5. A 67-year-old woman, had an eight year history of depression, which had been treated with a variety of antidepressants and lithium. She was admitted to psychiatric hospital because of her inability to function, memory impairment, disorientation and a suspicion that she was suffering from dementia. Neuropsychological testing revealed significant cognitive impairment. Because of her history of depression, she was treated with antidepressants, including tranylcypramine, with little improvement. In fact, her overall condition appeared to be worsening.

Additional stresses included severe marital discord, the couple having a 40 year history of a hostile-dependent relationship. The patient's husband refused to come to the hospital for an interview with the social worker. Because of her failure to respond, the team decided to take her off all medications and to give her as much therapeutic support as possible. Gradually her cognitive impairment and general functioning began to improve, to the point where it was possible to discharge her from hospital, with plans for her to attend a day care program. At the time of discharge there was no evidence of cognitive impairment and her only medication was lorazepam 1 mg at night when necessary. Follow-up included referral for psychotherapy and marital therapy. She subsequently maintained her progress although she experienced episodic anxiety and panic attacks particularly when she and her husband had a major quarrel.

It is not clear whether this woman's recovery was related to the support and lack of stress in the hospital environment or to the discontinuation of medications which might have been contributing to her cognitive impairment. A most critical aspect in the therapy of such patients involves the attempt to alter the system or environment in which the person lives and functions. This can involve such diverse interventions as family therapy, respite care and day care or other support services.

There have been few systematic studies of psychotic symptoms in association with dementia. One study found that 18% of 377 patients with primary dementia developed paranoid symptoms (Larsson, Sjogren and Jacobson, 1963). It has been suggested that when paranoia is present, the delusions tend to be poorly systematized and loosely held (Cummings 1985). Such delusions are often directly related to memory impairment for example, the person who loses possessions and then attributes this loss to theft. The more severely impaired patients are generally unable to give a

clear history of the experience themselves, so one tends to rely on
reports from staff or family members. The staff may often report
hallucinations, although it may be difficult, at times, to differentiate
illusions or delusions from true hallucinations.

Because of the loss of ability to process information, loss of insight
and language functions, and the inability to communicate, patients with
moderate to severe dementia are often incompetent to make decisions about
their own care. Consequently, significant ethical and moral questions
arise, for example, when such a patient absolutely refuses to eat, or
physically attacks other patients or staff. It is, of course, necessary
to involve and support families in making the difficult decisions which
must be considered.

Apart from depression and psychosis, there are a whole host of other
behaviours which may occur in conjunction with dementia. These include
verbal or physical aggressiveness, oppositional behaviour, wandering,
agitation and restlessness, belligerence, importuning, withdrawal and
refusal to eat. It is often these behavioural problems which cause the
greatest difficulty for caregivers. In a study of patients with mild
Alzheimer's disease, passive, agitated and "self-centred" behavioural
changes were noted on initial evaluation in two-thirds, one-third and
one-third of subjects, respectively. Over a 50-month follow-up period,
the percentage of patients who exhibited agitated and self-centred
behaviours doubled. The percentage of subjects who demonstrated all three
behavioural changes increased from 11% to over 50% when the dementia had
became severe (Rubin, Morris and Berg, 1987).

Case No.6. A 77-year-old widow was referred for a psychogeriatric
assessment because of her poor memory and decreasing ability to care
for herself. She lived in a small, totally unkempt, apartment and was
severely neglectful of her personal hygiene and grooming. She only
ate "junk food" and had an insatiable appetite for sweets. Her
husband had died of cancer 6 years earlier. Her only child, a son,
had died about 15 years before and his wife and children had
emigrated. Her nephew described increasing loss of memory, apathy
and depression in recent years.

The patient presented as timid, anxious, smelling of urine, talking in
a monotone and had some dyskinetic movements of her mouth. She was
disoriented to time and place, had very poor short-term memory and
decreased attention and calculation abilities. She scored 16 out of
30 on a Folstein mini-mental state exam. A diagnosis of moderate
dementia, most likely of the Alzheimer's type, was made.

One year later she was admitted to a nursing home and psychiatric evaluation was again requested because of agitated bahaviour. The staff described her constant questions, such as "what time is lunch?" or "who will come and get me?". She could not be reassured. At times, particularly when alone, she would talk to herself or her clothes, saying for example, "Go away pants!", leading the staff to think that she might be hallucinating. Sometimes she would talk gibberish and would change the tone of her voice so that it sounded like that of a man. The effect was of 2 people engaged in conversation. The other residents and some staff members were quite frightened by this. Several neuroleptics, including haloperidol (0.5 mg tid) and thioridazine (up to 10mg tid) were tried. However, she improved most on perphenazine, 4mg bid, which greatly decreased her agitation. Staff were encouraged to increase her attendance at activity programs and to give her a written schedule of her activities. Behavioural strategies to reinforce adaptive behaviour were also introduced. It appeared that these combined treatment strategies were responsible for the improvement in her condition.

This case demonstrates a number of the unusual and, at times, bizarre behaviours that can occur in patients with dementia. In this situation the patient's behaviours were distressing to others, and because of this she was shunned by her fellow residents, leading to further isolation, loneliness and agitation. Management of these behaviours often incorporates a variety of integrated approaches. The caregivers should always be involved in the planning of strategies to control these behaviours.

In patients with multi-infarct dementia there may be findings of both a cortical and sub-cortical nature. Psychomotor retardation and emotional lability are frequently present. This makes the diagnosis of depression even more problematic in these patients. The sub-cortical symptoms may include extreme slowness, depression and apathy.

Case No.7. A 78-year-old, married, semi-retired business man, with two children, was referred because of depression. He had developed some gait difficulty and had been seen by many neurologists accompanied by an extraordinary number of investigations. The only significant findings were some minor focal neurological abnormalities, most likely representing a small lacunar infarct. He was unable to focus on any issues apart from his declining physical state. His walking had become more difficult and his balance had deteriorated. There was definite evidence of cognitive impairment with decreased attention and short-term memory. The working diagnosis was multi-infarct dementia.

There was a family history of multiple losses in World War II. The
patient did not tolerate tricyclic antidepressants but there was
reduced anxiety on alprazolam (0.25mg tid). He constantly insisted
that something had to be done, that he could not continue to live like
this. He felt that there had to be some cure for his condition.
Despite numerous attempts to reassure him, he and his wife convinced
his family to organize visits to further specialists. He was admitted
to a geriatric psychiatric day hospital program to offer support and
increased help to his family. However, after a short period of time
in the program the family arranged an admission to yet another
hospital.

As this case illustrates, families and patients themselves may find it
extremely difficult to accept certain physical symptoms and
irreversible dysfunction. There may be denial and unrealistic
expectations about a magical cure. In such situations the failure to
reach acceptance impairs the ability to grieve for the losses. The
end result is often an iatrogenic complication, as more tests are
performed and more drugs are prescribed. The "shopping for a cure"
syndrome may lead to a lack of continuity of care. As a result the
patient and family may not receive much-needed support and consistent
medical care.

Huntington's Disease

Huntington's disease is an autosomal dominant, inherited disorder,
with a prevalence rate of between five and ten per 100,000 in the
population. The disease is characterized by a variety of involuntary and
abnormal movements of the body, dementia and psychiatric symptoms,
including depression, mania and psychosis. It is on occasion misdiagnosed
as either Parkinson's disease or schizophrenia. Huntington who described
the disorder in 1872 realized that patients frequently developed
"insanity" with a tendency towards suicide. Although the disorder most
frequently presents between the ages of 20 and 50, the onset has been
reported in old age. Studies have shown that up to 41% of patients have
suffered, at some time, from a major affective disorder (Folstein, Abbott,
Chaise, Jensen, and Folstein, 1983). Patients sometimes develop auditory
hallucinations or delusions (usually paranoid), although these symptoms
are not typical of the majority of cases. In Folstein's study, only 2 of
88 patients actually met DSM-III criteria for schizophrenia.

The neurological features of the disease include choreic movements,
occasionally hemichorea affecting one half of the body, and extrapyramidal signs. Cognitive impairment occurs, but is characterized by a
relative sparing of memory and orientation. Focal signs such as

dysphasia, apraxia and agnosia are rarely seen. However, there is apathy, slowed thinking, word finding difficulty and impaired judgement (McHugh and Folstein 1975; Wexler 1979). It is believed that many of these features relate to "subcortical dementia". Explosive irritability and aggression have also been described as frequent occurrences in this disease.

Studies suggest that suicide is a particularly common cause of death. One study of 102 patients, found that 10 attempted suicide and 13 self-mutilation. In addition, 19 were alcoholics and 18 had criminal convictions (Dewhurst, Oliver and McKnight, 1970). Another study found that suicide accounted for 7% of deaths in non-hospitalized patients (Reed and Chandler 1958). Perhaps one of the most harrowing aspects of the disease is the knowledge that one's children have a 50% chance of being afflicted with the same disorder. One might certainly postulate that resulting guilt might lead to the particularly high rate of depression and suicide.

The disease is caused by degeneration of the basal ganglia particularly the caudate nuclei. There is also marked atrophy of the frontal lobes with dilatation of the ventricular system, especially the frontal horns. Biochemical studies reveal reduced levels of gamma-aminobutyric acid (GABA) and low levels of choline acetyl-transferase (Perry, Hansen, and Kloster, 1973).

Motor Neurone Disease

Motor neurone disease, also referred to as amyotrophic lateral sclerosis usually has its onset between the ages of 50 and 70. The disease often begins with atrophy of the small muscles of the hand. Subsequently, the weakness progresses to involve the arms and legs and there is associated spasticity, particularly in the legs. There is a combination of upper and lower motor neuron signs and there may be an associated bulbar palsy. Emotional lability with pathological laughing and crying is not uncommon. The course is generally progressive, with most patients surviving for 2-3 years, although sometimes longer. Death usually results from bulbar involvement or respiratory failure secondary to weakness of the muscles of respiration. Psychiatric sequelae are not especially common in this disease, although depression, probably as a reactive phenomenon, certainly does occur. In an interesting study by Brown and Mueller (1970), in which 10 patients were carefully studied, there was a remarkable absence of depression. There appeared to be a great deal of psychological denial. The authors suggested that the premorbid personality of these patients was characteristically that of a pattern of mastery over their life and a tendency to exclude unpleasant feelings from conscious awareness.

Case No.8. A 73-year-old man, with a one year history of motor neurone disease, was referred because of depression. He was a bright, intelligent, articulate man who had been a successful businessman and active community member. He was philosophical and knowledgeable about his disease process but had thought through clear plans for suicide. He had decided that if the disease progressed to the point where he could no longer walk or glean pleasure from life, this would signal a natural point to end his life. He had periodic feelings of depression and was appropriately tearful when discussing his illness and his feelings. He had been treated with an antidepressant (imipramine 50 mg, hs) over the previous year and found it somewhat helpful. He had also been seeing a psychologist for supportive psychotherapy.

Subsequently, because of his wife's deteriorating health, he was unable to care for himself and was hospitalized in a long-term care unit. Despite a gradual deterioration of his condition, he was still mobile six months after the initial consultation. He had become an active and well-liked member of the hospital community and his extroverted, gregarious personality had helped him to form many new friendships. He seemed to offer a great deal of support to other patients with chronic disease. His condition did gradually deteriorate and he became wheelchair-bound. He died of respiratory complications.

This case raises the issue of rational suicide, and whether psychiatric intervention should be highly aggressive or essentially supportive in the care of patients with rapidly progressive illnesses, such as motor neurone disease. This man also demonstrated that zest for life, vitality and altruism, can continue in the face of an uncertain future.

Other Neurological Diseases

Cerebral tumours usually present with physical symptoms, however, occasionally, the first symptoms consist of emotional or behavioural changes. Studies of patients with tumours have found that psychological symptoms tend to occur in between half and three-quarters of patients (Keschner, Bender and Strauss, 1938; Hecaen and Ajuriaguerra 1956). Lishman (1978) makes the point that a variety of factors may influence the development of symptoms. These include raised intracranial pressure, the nature of the tumour, the rapidity of its growth and its location. He also makes the point that in patients with a special genetic predisposition to mental disorder the tumour may act as a precipitating factor only.

Alcoholic brain disease is important to consider in the elderly. The acute disorder of Wernicke's encephalopathy and the more chronic sequel, Korsakoff's psychosis are both found in the elderly. This condition is generally considered to be related to thiamine deficiency. The majority of patients with the acute illness develop the long-term amnestic condition (Victor, Adams and Collins, 1971). Victor et al observed the following frequency of signs in Wernicke's encephalopathy; mental abnormalities (90%), ocular abnormalities, including nystagmus and palsies (96%), ataxia (87%), peripheral neuropathy (82%), malnutrition (84%), and the abstinence syndrome (13%). They described the commonest mental abnormalities as a quiet, global confusion. At times there was evidence of mild delirium. Follow-up revealed that 84% developed the typical amnestic syndrome, and of those patients with Korsakoff's psychosis a quarter recovered completely, half showed some recovery, and there was no improvement in the others. Confabulation was found to be common, particularly early in the disorder, but was not always present.

Other vitamin deficiency disorders have been linked to psychiatric disorders. Certain psychiatric presentations such as depression, paranoia and organic mental syndromes may be associated with vitamin B12 deficiency (Zucker, Livingstone, Nakra and Clayton, 1981). There has also been some suggestion that low folate levels are common in depressed patients (Carney, 1967; Reynolds, Preece, Baily and Coppen, 1970).

COPING WITH NEUROPSYCHIATRIC ILLNESS

Having reviewed specific associations between psychiatric disorders and the common neurological diseases of the elderly, it is useful to consider some of the psychological mechanisms whereby individuals cope with such problems. There have been a variety of definitions of the term coping. Lazarus (1966) defines coping, simply, as the strategies one uses to deal with threat. Coping may also be described as the course of action that one takes in response to a problem, to bring about relief, reward, quiescence and equilibrium. It is considered to be a dynamic process of action which includes cognitive and behavioural activity and the use of psychological defense mechanisms. The ultimate aim of coping is mastery, control or resolution. Coping tasks may be required, not only to deal with the physical effects of an illness and associated loss of functioning, but, also, with changes in perception, for example, anxiety associated with thoughts of further deterioration or impending death, as well as internal psychic phenomenon such as threatened body image or fears of alterations in family relationships.

There has been some work on age-related changes in coping. Vaillant (1977) and Pfeiffer (1977) suggest that individuals become more effective and realistic in their coping mechanisms as they age. They suggest that there is less dependence on immature mechanisms such as projection and acting out, and more use of mature mechanisms such as altruism, humour and suppression. Conversely, Gutmann (1974) suggests that, as people age, they move from active mastery to more passive modes and ultimately to a reliance on magical modes. It has also been suggested that people of all ages cope similarly when they are dealing with similar forms of stress, but that the forms of stress change over the life course. Folkman (1986) reported that older subjects use more distancing and positive reappraisal than younger subjects. Breznitz (1986) has suggested that the very term, "coping strategy", is a misnomer. He proposes that the majority of individuals under stressful situations revert towards stereotypic behaviour, rather than developing effective coping strategies.

Miller (1983) has described a typology of the coping tasks of chronically ill adults. The task categories are: maintaining a sense of normalcy; modifying daily routines and adjusting life style; obtaining knowledge and skill for continuing self-care; adjusting to altered social relationships; grieving over losses concomitant with chronic illness; dealing with role change; handling physical discomfort; complying with prescribed regimens; confronting the inevitability of one's own death; dealing with social stigmata of illness or disability; maintaining a feeling of being in control; and maintaining hope, despite an uncertain or downward course of health.

Specific coping strategies can be divided into "approach" and "avoidance". Approach strategies include seeking information, enhancing one's spiritual life, using methods of self-distraction, sharing feelings and developing specific routines of physical relaxation and exercise. Avoidance strategies include the use of denial, minimizing symptoms and withdrawal. Weisman (1979) described good copers as resourceful, not rigid and characterized by the fact that they avoid denial and take action based on confronting reality; they redefine problems into solvable forms, considering alternatives, maintain open communications, seek help and accept support, and ultimately maintain hope.

Kimball (1979) describes the tasks of coping with illness and contrasts the patient's tasks with those of the staff, who care for the patient (see table 3). He makes the important point that it is often crucial to accept dependency and to give oneself permission to be ill. It is also vital for the staff to give permission to the patient to be ill and to permit normal emotional reactions. It may at times be easier for staff to accept the normal behaviour of a sick person when that person is elderly in comparison to the younger patient, with whom younger staff members identify more easily.

Virtually all elderly people must cope with multiple losses as they and their loved ones experience a deterioration in their health, the loss of friends through illness and death, the loss of independence, control and roles. While many elderly people are able to continue to thrive and enjoy life, many of those patients who suffer from neuropsychiatric disorders have to cope with considerable loss. Frequently, the associated cognitive impairments diminish their capacity to cope in an efficient manner. Former coping mechanisms and the individual's premorbid personality, play a major role in determining how the person actually copes. Ultimately, if the individual is to avoid despair he must be able to integrate the events of his life and to reach some form of overall acceptance (Erikson, 1959).

CONCLUSION

The common neurological diseases of the elderly, particularly the dementias, stroke and Parkinson's disease are all associated with changes in emotion, thinking and behaviour. The resulting neuropsychiatric syndromes are of a diverse nature. The cases described above, illustrate the numerous factors which must be considered by the clinician and treatment team when caring for such patients. Management decisions may involve the consideration of a variety of factors, including the nature of the brain disease and its likely course, superimposed organic mental disorders, associated cognitive abilities, strengths and impairments, current medications including psychotropic medications, the premorbid personality, psychiatric history and family history, and family and individual psychodynamics. Moral, ethical and legal dilemmas are frequent and must be taken into account when making clinical decisions. The individual's coping mechanisms should be considered in relation to the normal developmental tasks of aging.

Whereas the desire to understand behaviour in simple terms is compelling, it behooves us to be ultra-cautious in our attempts to be "all knowing". It is tempting to simply attribute a particular emotion or behaviour to specific and localized brain disease or to certain alterations in neurochemistry. This model is unsatisfactory. It does not fit with our understanding of the mind and is absurdly reductionistic. Such approaches may be appealing to those professionals who have trouble accepting the uncertainties and ambiguities that remain a necessary part of medical-psychiatric practice.

Whether in the institution or in the community, optimal care requires an integrated, truly multi-disciplinary approach. The authors of this book discuss various forms of intervention, all of which have an important

TABLE 3: THE TASKS OF ILLNESS. From Kimball, C.P. (1979). Reactions to Illness: The Acute Phase. Psych Clinics of N. America (2) 307-319

Phase of Illness	Staff	Patient
I. Acute	1. Permission to be ill	Accepts partial dependent position based upon acceptance of illness
	2. Permission to ventilate	Talks about fears, sadness, anger
	3. Accepts ventilation	Tries various defenses
	4. Accepts and helps shape appropriate defenses	Accepts therapist's suggestions and encouragement
II. Convalescent	5. Accepts patient's convalescence	Conservation-withdrawal
	6. Allows patient to continue to grieve	Uses increasingly sophisticated mechanisms of defense
	7. Exhorts patient to self-care	Accepts self-care
III. Rehabilitation	8. Supports positive coping & adaptive strategies	Prepares self for the event of the home-coming

role to play in the care of these patients. The relative merits of these different forms of treatment are still uncertain. Much work lies ahead in our attempts to understand the potential benefits, as well as the possible pitfalls, of integrating these differing management approaches.

REFERENCES

Alexander, M.P., Geschwind, N. (1984). Dementia in the elderly. In Albert, M.L. (ed). Clinical Neurology of Aging. New York: Oxford University Press.

American Psychiatric Association, (1980). Diagnostic and Statistical Manual of Mental Disorders. (third edition). Washington, D.C.: American Psychiatric Association.

American Psychiatric Association, (1987). Diagnostic and Statistical Manual of Mental Disorders. (third edition - revised). Washington, D.C.: American Psychiatric Association.

Angst, J. (1986). The epidemiology of late-onset depression. In Kielholz, P., Adams, C. (eds.). The Elderly Person as a Patient. Köln: Deutcher Ärzte-Verlag.

Berrios, G.E. (1987). The nosology of the dementias: An Overview. In Pitt, B. (ed.) Dementia. Edinburgh: Churchill Livingstone.

Breznitz, S. (1986). Are there coping strategies? In McHugh, S., Vallis, T.M. (eds.). Illness Behaviour: A Multidisciplinary Model. New York: Plenum, 325-329.

Birkmayer W., Reiderer, P. (1975). Responsibility of extrastriatal areas for the appearance of psychotic symptoms (clinical and biochemical human post-mortem findings). J. Neural Transm. 37, 175-182.

Bleuler, E.P. (1951). Textbook of Psychiatry. New York: Dover Publications.

Brown, W.A., Mueller, P.S. (1970). Psychological function in individuals with amyotrophic lateral sclerosis. Psychosom. Med. 32, 141-152.

Carney, M.W.P. (1967). Serum folate values in 423 psychiatric patients. Brit. Med. J., 512-516.

Carroll, B.J. (1976). Limbic system-adrenal cortex regulation in depression and schizophrenia. Psychosom. Med. 38, 106-121.

Celesia, G.G., Wanamaker W.M. (1972). Psychiatric disturbances in Parkinson's disease. Diseases of the Nervous System 33, 577-583.

Chapman, L.F., Wolff, H.G. (1959). The cerebral hemispheres and the highest integrative functions of man. Arch Neurol. 1, 357-424.

Conn, D.K. (1986). Managing neuropsychiatric disorders in the elderly. Perspectives in Geriatrics. 2, 46-56.

Cummings, J. (1988). Organic psychosis. Psychosomatics, 29, 16-26.

Cummings, J.L. (1985). Clinical neuropsychiatry. Orlando: Grune and Stratton.

Cummings, J.L., Mendez, M.F. (1984). Secondary mania with focal cerebrovascular lesions. Am. J. Psychiatry. 141, 1084-1087.

Davison, K., Bagley, C.R. (1969). Schizophrenia-like psychoses associated with organic disorders of the central nervous system: A review of the literature. In Herrington, R.N. (ed.) Current Problems In Neuropsychiatry. British J. Psych. Special Publication No.4. Ashford, Kent: Headley Brothers.

Dewhurst, K., Oliver, J.E., McKnight, A.L. (1970). Socio-psychiatric consequences of Huntington's disease. Br. J. Psychiatry. 116, 255-258.

Eisdorfer, C., Busse, E., Cohen, L. (1959). The WAIS performance of an aged sample: the relationship between verbal and performance I.Q.s. J. Gerontol. 14, 197-201.

Engel, G. (1977). The need for a new medical model: a challenge for biomedicine. Science, 196, 129-136.

Erikson, E.H. (1959). Identity and the life cycle. Psychological Issues, Monograph 1. New York: International Universities Press.

Erikson, T.C. (1945). Erotomania (nymphomania) as expressions of cortical epileptiform discharge. Arch. Neurol. Psychiat. 53, 226-231.

Fibiger, H.C. (1984). The neurobiological substrates of depression in Parkinson's disease: a hypothesis. Can. J. Neurol. Sci. 11(I Suppl). 105-107.

Folkman, S. (1986). Coping over the life span. In McHugh, S., Vallis, T.M. (eds.). Illness Behaviour: A Multidisciplinary Model. New York: Plenum, 321-324.

Folstein, M.F., Maiberger, R., McHugh, P.R. (1977). Mood disorder as a specific complication of stroke. J. Neurol, Neurosurg. Psychiatry. 40, 1018-1020.

Folstein, S.E., Abbott, M.H., Chaise, G.A., Jensen, B.A., Folstein, M.F. (1983). The association of affective disorder with Huntington's disease in a case series and in families. Psychol. Med. 13, 537-542.

Freemon, F.R. (1976). Evaluation of patients with progressive intellectual deterioration. Arch. Neurol., 33, 658-659.

Gotham, A.M., Brown, R.G., Marsden, C.D. (1986). Depression in parkinson's disease: a quantitative and qualitative analysis. J. Neurol. Neurosurg. Psychiatry, 49, 381-389.

Gutmann, D.L. (1974). The country of old men: cross-cultural studies in the psychology of later life. In Levine, R.L. (ed.) Culture and Personality: Contemporary Readings. New York: Aldine.

Hagnell, O., Lanke, J., Porsman, B., Ohman, R., Ojesjo, L. (1983). Current trends in the incidence of senile and multi-infarct dementia. Archives of Psychiatry and Neurological Sciences. 233, 423-438.

Hécaen, H., Ajuriaguerra, J. (1956). Troubles Mentaux Au Cours Des Tumeurs Intracraniennes. Paris: Masson.

Henderson, A.S. (1987). Alzheimer's disease: epidemiology. In Pitt, B. (ed.). Dementia. Edinburgh: Churchill Livingstone.

Henry, J.P. (1987). Psychological factors and coronary heart disease. Holistic Medicine. 2, 119-132.

Henry, J.P., Stephens, P.M. (1977). Stress, Health and the Social Environment - A Sociobiological Approach to Medicine. New York: Springer-Verlag.

Hochanadel, G., Kaplan, E. (1984). Neuropsychology of normal aging. In Albert, M.L. (ed.). Clinical Neurology Of Aging. New York: Oxford University Press.

Hodgins, E. (1964). Episode: Report on the Accident Inside My Skull. New York: Antheneum.

Hoehn, M.M., Yahr, M.D. (1967). Parkinsonism: onset, progression and mortality. Neurology, 17, 427-442.

Horn, S. (1974). Some psychological factors in Parkinsonism. J. Neurol, Neurosurg and Psychiatry, 37, 27-31.

House, A. (1987). Mood disorders after stroke: review of the evidence. Intl. J. Geriatric Psychiatry. 2, 211-221.

Jacques, S. (1979). Brain stimulation and reward: "pleasure centres" after twenty-five years. Neurosurgery, 5, 277-283.

Keschner, M., Bender, M.B., Strauss, I. (1938). Mental symptoms associated with brain tumour: a study of 530 verified cases. J.A.M.A., 110, 714-718.

Kiloh, L.G. (1961). Pseudo-dementia. Acta Psychiatr. Scand. 37, 336-351.

Kimball, C.P. (1979). Reactions to illness: the acute phase. Psychiatric Clinics of N. America, 2, 307-319.

Klawans, H.L., Moskovitz, C., Nausieda, P.A. Weiner, W.J. (1979). Levodopa-induced dopaminergic hypersensitivity in the pathogenesis of psychiatric and neurological disorders. Int. J. Neurol. 13, 225.

Klüver, H., Bucy, P.C. (1939). Preliminary analysis of the temporal lobes in monkeys. Arch. Neurol. Psychiat. 42, 979-1000.

Knesevich, J.W., Martin, R.L., Berg, L., Danziger, W. (1983). Preliminary report on affective symptoms in the early stages of senile dementia of the Alzheimer type. Am. J. Psychiatry. 140, 233-35.

Kral, V.A. (1983). The relationship between senile dementia (Alzheimer type) and depression. Can. J. Psychiatry, 28, 304-306.

Krauthammer, C., Klerman, G.L. (1978). Secondary mania: manic syndromes associated with antecedent physical illness or drugs. Arch. Gen. Psychiatry. 135, 1333-1339.

Larsson, T., Sjogren, T., Jacobson, G. (1963). Senile dementia. Acta Psychiatr. Scand. (suppl). 167, 1-259.

Lashley, K.S. (1929). Brain Mechanisms and Intelligence. Chicago: University of Chicago Press.

Lazarus, R. (1966). Psychological Stress and the Coping Process. New York: McGraw-Hill.

Levine, D.N., Finklestein, S. (1982). Delayed psychosis after right temporoparietal stroke or trauma: relation to epilepsy. Neurology, 32, 267-273.

Lipowski, Z.J. (1981). Organic mental disorders: their history and classification with special reference to DSM-III. In Miller, N.E., Cohen, G.D. (eds.) Clinical Aspects of Alzheimer's Disease and Senile Dementia. New York: Raven Press.

Lipowski, Z.J. (1984). Organic mental disorders - an American perspective. Br. J. Psychiatry. 144, 542-546.

Lipsey, J.R., Robinson R.G., Pearlson, G.D., Rao, K., Price, T.R. (1984). Nortriptyline treatment of post-stroke depression: a double-blind treatment trial. Lancet 1, 297-300.

Lishman, W. (1978). Organic Psychiatry. Oxford: Blackwell Scientific Publications.

Lishman, W. (1987). Organic Psychiatry. 2nd Edition. Oxford: Blackwell Scientific Publications.

Lowy, L. (1986). The implication of demographic trends as they affect the elderly. J. Geriatr. Psychiatry. 19, 149-174.

Madden, J.J., Luhan, J.A., Kaplan, L.A., Manfredi, H.M. (1952). Nondementing psychoses in older persons. J.A.M.A., 150, 1567-1570.

Marsden, C.D., Harrison, M.J.G. (1972). Outcome of investigation of patients with presenile dementia. Br. Med. J. 2, 249-252.

Mayeux, R., Stern, Y., Cote, L., Williams, J.B. (1984). Altered serotonin metabolism in depressed patients with Parkinson's disease. Neurology. 34, 642-646.

McAllister, T.W., Price, T.R.P. (1982). Severe depressive pseudodementia with and without dementia. Am. J. Psychiatry. 139, 626-629.

McHugh, P.R., Folstein, M.F. (1975). Psychiatric syndromes of Huntington's chorea. In Benson, D.F., Blumer, D. (eds.). Psychiatric Aspects Of Neurologic Disease. New York: Grune and Stratton.

McHugh, S., Vallis, M. (1986). Illness behaviour: operationalization of the biopsychosocial model. In McHugh, S., Vallis, M. (eds.) Illness Behaviour - A Multidisciplinary Model. New York: Plenum Press.

Mesulam, M.M. (1979). Acute behavioural derangements without hemiplegia in cerebrovascular accidents. Primary Care. 6, 813-826.

Miller, J.F. (1983). Coping with chronic illness. In Coping With Chronic Illness: Overcoming Powerlessness. Philadelphia: F.A. Davis.

Mortimer, J.A., Schuman, L.M., French, L.R. (1981). Epidemiology of dementing illness. In Mortimer, J.A., Schuman, L.M. (eds.) The Epidemiology of Dementia. New York: Oxford University Press.

Moskovitz, C., Moses, H. 3d, Klawans, H.L. (1978). Levodopa-induced psychosis: a kindling phenomenon. Am. J. Psychiatry, 135, 669-675.

Murray, G.B., Shea, V.A., Conn, D.K. (1986). Electroconvulsive therapy for post-stroke depression. J. Clin. Psychiatry, 47, 258-260.

National Center for Health Statistics (1979). The National Nursing Home Survey: 1977 Summary for the United States. Vital and Health Statistics, Serial 13, Number 43. Government Printing Office: Washington, D.C.

Nott, P.N., Fleminger, J.J. (1975). Presenile dementia: the difficulties of early diagnosis. Acta Psychiatr. Scand., 51, 210-217.

Papez, J.W. (1937). A proposed mechanism of emotion. Arch. Neurol. Psychiat. 38, 725-743.

Perry, T.L., Hansen, S., Kloster, M. (1973). Huntington's chorea: deficiency of gamma-aminobutyric acid in the brain. N. Eng. J. Med. 288, 337-342.

Pfeiffer, E. (1977). Psychopathology and social pathology. In Birren, J.E., Schaie K.W., (eds.). Handbook Of The Pathology Of Aging. New York: Van Nostrand Reinhold.

Pincus, J.H., Tucker, G.J. (1978). Behavioural Neurology. New York: Oxford University Press.

Platt, D. (1986). Biological and medical aspects of aging. In Kielholz, P., Adams, C. (eds.) The Elderly Person As A Patient. Köln: Deutscher Arzte-Verlag.

Plum, F. (1979). Dementia: an approaching epidemic. Nature, 279, 372-373.

Reding, M.J., Orto, L.A., Winter, S.A., Fortuna, I.M., Di Ponte, P., McDowell, F.H. (1986). Antidepressant therapy after stroke: a double-blind study. Arch. Neurol., 43, 763-765.

Reed, T.E., Chandler, J.H. (1958). Huntington's chorea in Michigan I: demography and genetics. Am. J. Human Genetics. 10, 201-225.

Reeves, A.G., Plum, F. (1969). Hyperphagia, rage and dementia accompanying a ventromedial hypothalamic neoplasm. Arch Neurol. 20, 616-624.

Reifler, B.V., Larson, E., Hanley, R. (1982). Coexistence of cognitive impairment and depression in geriatric outpatients. Am. J. Psychiatry. 139, 623-626.

Reynolds, E.H., Preece, J.M., Bailey, J., Coppen, A. (1970). Folate deficiency in depressive illness. Br. J. Psychiatry. 117, 287-292.

Robins, A. (1976). Are stroke patients more depressed than other disabled subjects? J. Chronic Dis. 29, 479-482.

Robinson, R.G. (1979). Differential behavioural and biochemical effects of right and left hemispheric cerebral infarction in the rat. Science. 205, 707-710.

Robinson, R.G., Lipsey, J.R., Kolla-Wilson, K. Bolduc, P.L., Pearlson, G.D., Rao, K., Price, T. (1985). Mood disorders in left-handed stroke patients. Am. J. Psychiatry. 142, 1424-1429.

Robinson, R.G., Kubos, K.L., Starr, L.B., Rao, K., Price, T.R. (1983). Mood changes in stroke patients: relationship to lesion location. Compr. Psychiatry. 24, 555-566.

Robinson, R.G., Starr, L.B., Kubos, K.L., Price, T.R. (1983). A two year longitudinal study of post-stroke mood disorders: findings during the initial evaluation. Stroke. 14, 736-741.

Robinson, R.G., Starr, L.B., Price, T.R. (1984). A two year longitudinal study of mood disorders following stroke: prevalence and duration at six months follow-up. Br. J. Psychiatry. 144, 256-262.

Ron, M.A., Toone, B.K., Garralda, M.E., Lishman, W.A. (1979). Diagnostic accuracy in presenile dementia. Brit. J. Psychiatry. 134, 161-168.

Rosenbaum, F., Harati, Y., Rolak, L., Freedman, M. (1987). Visual hallucinations in sane people: Charles Bonnet syndrome. J. Am. Geriatr. Soc. 35, 66-68.

Ross, E.D., Rush, J. (1981). Diagnosis and neuroanatomical correlates of depression in brain-damaged patients. Arch. Gen. Psychiatry. 38, 1344-1354.

Rubin, E.H., Morris, J.C., Berg, L. (1987). The progression of personality changes in senile dementia of the Alzheimer's type. J. Am. Geriatr. Soc. 35, 721-725.

Ruggieri, S., Stocchi, F., Denaro, A., Baronti, F., Agnoli, A. (1986). The role of Mao-b inhibitors in the treatment of Parkinson's disease. J. Neurol. Transm. 22 (suppl), 227-233.

Savage, G.H. (1890). Insanity And Allied Neuroses. London: Cassel and Co.

Shulman, K., Post, F. (1980). Bipolar affective disorder in old age. Br. J. Psychiatry. 136, 26-32.

Sim, M., Sussman, I. (1962). Alzheimer's disease: its natural history and differential diagnosis. J. Nerv. Ment. Dis. 134, 489-499.

Spitzer, R.L., Williams, J.B.W., Skodol, A.E. (1983). International Perspectives On DSM-III. Washington, D.C.: American Psychiatric Press, Inc.

Stedman's Medical Dictionary (1982). 24th Edition. Baltimore: Williams and Wilkins.

Strub, R.L., Black, F.W. (1981). Organic Brain Syndromes - An Introduction To Neurobehavioural Disorders. Philadelphia: F.A. Davis Company.

Taylor, A.E., Saint-Cyr, J.A., Lang, A.E., Kenny, F.T. (1986). Parkinson's disease and depression: a critical re-evaluation. Brain. 109, 279-292.

Torack, R.M. (1983). The early history of senile dementia, In Reisberg, B. (ed.) Alzheimer's Disease - The Standard Reference. New York: The Free Press.

Vaillant, G.E. (1977). Adaptation To Life. Boston: Little, Brown.

Victor, M., Adams, R.D., Collins, G.H. (1971). The Wernicke-Korsakoff Syndrome. Oxford: Blackwell Scientific Publications.

Wechsler, D. (1958). The Measurement And Appraisal Of Adult Intelligence, 4th Ed. Baltimore: Williams and Wilkins.

Weisman, A. (1979). Coping With Cancer. New York: McGraw-Hill.

Wells, C.E. (1979). Pseudodementia. Am. J. Psychiatry 136, 895-900.

Wexler, B.E. (1980). Cerebral laterality and psychiatry: a review of the literature. Am. J. Psychiatry. 137, 279-291.

Wexler, N.S. (1979). Perceptual-motor, cognitive, and emotional characteristics of persons at risk for huntington's disease. In Chase, T.N., Wexler, N.S., Barbeau, A. (eds.) Advances In Neurology, Vol.23; Huntington's Disease. New York: Raven Press.

Zucker, D.K., Livingstone, R.L., Nakra, R., Clayton, P.J. (1981). B_{12} Deficiency and psychiatric disorders: case report and literature review. Biol. Psychiatry. 16, 197-205.

CHAPTER 2

INVESTIGATION OF NEUROPSYCHIATRIC DISORDERS

Stuart A. Schneck, M.D.
University of Colorado
School of Medicine
Denver, Colorado

The cerebral disorders most likely to have psychiatric consequences in old age are dementia, Parkinson's disease and stroke.

DEMENTIA

Patients in whom dementia is suspected reach the physician in a number of ways. Least common is self-referral; much more frequent are referrals from family members, usually children, who begin to suspect a meaning to a persistent pattern of leaving the stove on, forgetting recent events and repeating questions just answered. Spouses are usually much more tolerant of this behaviour, because until quite recently it was considered an inevitable part of the aging process. Not so the children, who today are quite familiar with Alzheimer's disease and have matured in a culture which expects that for every diagnosis there is a treatment, if not a cure. Referrals are also quite commonly stimulated by employers or supervisors who notice evidence of impaired performance at work. Such patients often get to the physician at a much earlier age and stage of the illness than those whose life centers primarily about the home, and whose performance may be evaluated less critically.

The first thing that the physician must do is take a history. Has there been a persistent intellectual decline from the previous level? Has there been a decline of sufficient severity to interfere with the social and occupational activities of that person?

Sometimes patients can give quite a clear history of intellectual change, particularly those who start from a high level of functioning and

51

become aware early on of difficulty with tasks that were previously quite easy. However, in less sophisticated people or in those whose livelihood might be at stake, details suggestive of dementia may be hard to elicit or may even be denied. It is, therefore, often essential to obtain information from others, with the consent of the patient or the family or both, in order to obtain as complete a picture as possible of the intellect and behaviour of the patient. This is of extreme importance when one is assessing the competence of professional people, such as physicians or attorneys, to do their work.

In evaluating the patient, it is necessary to ascertain whether or not other neurological disorders have preceded or co-exist with dementia. Family history, the neurologic examination itself and laboratory tests will also enter into the diagnosis of these disorders. The list of possibilities is very long, but most important would be Parkinson's disease, Huntington's disease, progressive supranuclear palsy, multiple cerebral infarcts, multiple sclerosis, head trauma, exposure to toxins (of which alcohol and drugs are the most prominent), and AIDS. The last is becoming more common, and cases of dementia manifested by memory loss, poor judgement and apathy are occasionally seen before it is apparent that the disease is present.

After the history, the general and the basic neurological examination, it is necessary to assess the mental status of the patient. How intensively this is done depends on how clear the diagnosis of dementia appears to be. If the patient can give few details of his own history despite full consciousness, has significant difficulty following the directions in the examination, and has a history consistent with intellectual deterioration, not too much more testing of the mental status need be done. On the other hand, if the presence or absence of dementia is still uncertain, then a number of additional tests of mental status are needed to assess alertness, attention, orientation, short-term learning ability, language, writing and reading, recent memory and recall, calculation, abstract thinking, constructional ability, general knowledge, mood, and thought content. Mental status testing may range from such brief tests as those of Kokmen, Naessens, and Offord (1987) at the Mayo Clinic and the commonly used Mini-mental Status test of Folstein, Folstein, and McHugh (1975) to more elaborate ones that take from 40 to 60 minutes.

It is worth emphasizing that any form of mental status testing may be quite threatening to the patient. One should try to defuse the situation as much as possible by maintaining a friendly and nonjudgemental demeanor. The tests and the reasons for them should be explained simply, and the patient's agreement to them obtained. The patient can be warned that it is unlikely that he will get the correct answer to every one of the questions. Encouraging comments can be made when appropriate to indicate to the patient that at least some of the responses are quite good.

At this point, it should be clearer whether dementia is present, and whether or not it is progressive. The next step is to establish, if possible, the most likely diagnosis and whether it can be specifically treated. Clinical and pathological studies show that of those patients with dementia in the absence of head trauma, about 50-60 percent have Alzheimer's disease, about 10-15 percent have multi-infarct dementia, and 10-15 percent have a combination of these two disorders (Tomlinson, Blessed and Roth, 1970). The remainder have a variety of diagnoses which include normal pressure hydrocephalus; some infectious diseases such as chronic fungal infections, neurosyphilis and Creutzfeldt-Jacob disease; other degenerative diseases such as Pick's and diffuse Lewy body disease; metabolic and drug-induced disorders; and depression. Perhaps 2 to 8 percent of dementias still do not readily fit into convenient diagnostic categories. The clinical examination is quite likely to yield an accurate impression of the cause. Confirmation by laboratory tests is the next step.

These can be numerous and costly if not chosen judiciously. Most clinicians would order a blood count with differential and red cell indices, sedimentation rate, and a biochemical screening battery as part of a general survey. A blood VDRL should always be done. Vitamin B12, folate and thyroid screening tests can be selectively performed. Whether one needs an electrocardiogram; chest x-ray; a dexamethasone suppression test for depression; and urine studies for amino acids and heavy metals clearly depends on the specific case. The value of the electroencephalogram EEG) in dementia has been questioned because of its relative lack of specificity. It is a useful test to do in a dementia "work-up", for if it is normal or nearly so, it offers more support for a degenerative or depressive disorder than for a diagnosis with focal features such as tumour or stroke. An imaging test of some type is mandatory in the search for treatable lesions. The magnetic resonance scan (MR) is preferable to the uncontrasted computed tomographic scan (CT) since it provides much more information about neural tissue; but it is more costly and has the disadvantage of showing a variety of abnormalities in the white matter with which firm clinical-pathological correlations have yet to be made. These white matter abnormalities, called unidentified bright objects, or leuko-araiosis (Hachinski, Potter and Mersky, 1987), do not normally occur in people under 50 to 54 years old. Over this age, they occur with increasing frequency, appear related in many cases to the presence of hypertension, and do not correlate with Alzheimer's disease. Early pathological reports suggest the likelihood that they may represent areas of subclinical ischemic injury or focal areas of tissue shrinkage. In the absence of clinical information, one cannot from a CT or MR scan make a diagnosis of dementia based upon ventricular or subarachnoid enlargement unless the changes are extreme. Ventricular size normally increases between the ages of 65 and 90, as does the subarachnoid space, somewhat less in women than in men, and this makes it difficult to make absolute correlations with dementia. The observation from pneumoencephalography that gross enlargement of the third ventricle due to atrophy of the thalamus and hypothalamus, in the absence of obstruction, is often correlated with dementia seems to be confirmed by contemporary imaging. Brain volume loss seen on CT may be reversible in some cases and one must know a good deal about the clinical data before pronouncing an apparent atrophy irreversible. Such reversibility has been seen in chronic alcoholism, anorexia nervosa, Cushing's disease, and in patients on high doses of steroids and chemotherapy.

Should the spinal fluid be examined? Those who would do so in every case cite the occasional detection of malignancy or chronic fungal, syphilitic or other infection. This is very unlikely, and in older patients lumbar puncture can be reserved for those with a reasonable clinical suspicion of a positive result. In relatively young patients, the possibility of AIDS now favours universal spinal taps since dementia can occasionally occur before other clinical evidence of the disease. In the future lumbar punctures on all demented patients may be indicated, for there is reason to hope that a relatively specific spinal fluid test for Alzheimer's disease may be developed in the near future.

Neuropsychological tests are sometimes ordered. They no more make a diagnosis of Alzheimer's disease than do the imaging studies, but they often delineate a variety of areas of subclinical cerebral dysfunction. Some psychologists use a standard battery of tests in an invariable fashion for every clinical problem, for example, the Halstead-Reitan battery. Others are more selective and target their tests toward problem areas; but the tests often confirm the obvious and leave unanswered the clinically questionable. The use of neuropsychological tests should be selective and sparing. The Minnesota Multiphasic Personality Inventory (MMPI) may be more useful than the other psychological tests if it gives support to a diagnosis of depression. A psychiatric consultation may help to establish whether depression or dementia is the problem in some questionable cases. They often go hand-in-hand early in dementia. Sometimes a therapeutic trial of an antidepressant may be informative. Brain biopsy is rarely indicated for diagnosis since the yield in diffuse degenerative disease is quite small. In summary, the history and examination, blood count, sedimentation rate, serology, biochemical screens, EEG and either CT or MR scan should yield a correct diagnosis of dementia and its cause in 85 to 90 percent of cases (Katzman, 1986). In

Denver, Colorado, this evaluation would cost between $850 and $1,000. This may seem expensive, but finding even the occasional case of treatable dementia, may result in human and financial savings which far outweigh the cost. For the elderly patient at home this basic level of investigation is satisfactory. For the younger, employed patients in whom causation is less obvious, greater consideration would usually be given to the additional studies mentioned.

PARKINSON'S DISEASE

In Parkinson's disease, investigation is straight forward because except in rare instances it is neither needed nor readily available. This disorder is one of the few left in medicine which can nearly always be correctly diagnosed by history, observation of the patient, and a few corroborative manoeuvres to bring out tremor, test the integrity of certain postural reflexes and demonstrate rigidity and bradykinesia. Positron emission tomography (PET scanning) may prove to be a test which can be used early to validate a clinical diagnosis, but at the present time it is extremely expensive and is available only in a few centers. The main differential diagnoses are drug-induced extrapyramidal disease; the changes of age in the extrapyramidal system; and benign essential or familial tremor. In normal people, extrapyramidal signs and symptoms are presumably based on the loss of approximately 50 percent of the pigmented substantia nigra cells by age 80, and they usually progress much more slowly and with much less severity than Parkinson's disease. Exaggerated physiological tremors are for the most part action or intention tremors which are the reverse of the resting tremors of the Parkinsonian. These physiologic tremors may actually begin very early in life. Occasionally the diagnosis is difficult when the disease is focal or the signs partial. With observation over time the situation usually clarifies itself.

A true dementia is not uncommon in Parkinson's disease; the frequency has ranged from 25 to 80 percent in various studies (Lieberman, Dziatolowski and Kupersmith, 1979; Brown and Marsden, 1984; Mortimer, Christensen and Webster, 1985) but it is generally accepted that about half of Parkinsonian patients do show evidence of some dementia, occasionally quite significant. Usually these are the patients whose motor problems are quite severe. Whether the cognitive change is due to age, medication or an associated pathological process acting singly or together is not known. In addition, depression, which can affect cognitive processes, is common and long-lasting in Parkinson's disease, probably even more so than in Alzheimer's disease. The usual pattern of development is that Parkinson's disease is diagnosed first; depression follows as the patient struggles to cope with motor problems; and then there is the onset of forgetfulness, occasional confusion, mental slowness, concrete thinking, lack of initiative, hallucinations, and delusions. This type of dementia has been called subcortical (Cummings and Benson, 1983) in contrast with the cortical dementia of Alzheimer's disease, in which patients are more alert but language disturbances are more striking. In many of the patients with Parkinson's disease and dementia, there are neuropathological features of both Parkinson's and Alzheimer's diseases, including neurofibrillary tangles, neuritic plaques and degeneration of the basal forebrain nuclei. Neuronal loss appears to affect not only dopaminergic innervation of the cerebral cortex but noradrenergic and cholinergic systems as well. In other patients it is harder to define why the dementia has occurred. In relatively few patients the dementia may precede the parkinsonian features, and one may at autopsy find evidence of diffuse Lewy body deposition in cortical, limbic and subcortical neurons.

There is little point in undertaking extensive investigations for the cause of dementia in the typical Parkinsonian patient especially if his course has been followed for years. Careful attention to the least expensive of all neurological tests, namely the neurological examination, and possibly an uncontrasted CT scan, especially if the patient has been falling, are the only things that seem necessary. Attempting to reduce the dose of medication may alleviate the intellectual difficulty somewhat and can be thought of as a therapeutic test. It is important to take this dementia seriously and to demonstrate one's concern to the patient and family with adequate discussion and explanation in order to provide additional emotional support in what is already a difficult situation due to the Parkinson's disease itself.

ISCHEMIC STROKE

For the patient with mental problems thought possibly related to ischemic events, particularly those which reverse completely or nearly so in a few days, a cerebral angiogram is mandatory unless specific contraindications exist in a particular patient. Whether the angiogram should be intra-arterial or intravenous, and whether vascular studies, coagulation tests, CT or MR, electrocardiography and echocardiography are also needed depends on the individual case. It must be remembered that the reason for doing these studies is to arrive at a diagnosis of a specific cause in order to minimize its effect in the future and so save other areas of brain that are at risk. In patients with completed strokes, extensive study may yield little of practical importance, and the facts of the particular case must determine the need for investigation.

While intravenous digital angiography is simpler to perform, less risky and cheaper than conventional selective intra-arterial cerebral angiography, it yields less detailed information. It is nonselective, limited in its viewing planes and often does not show smaller vessels very well. Therefore, if a patient truly has had an ischemic attack, conventional angiography is needed. Noninvasive studies, of which carotid ultrasound is the prime example, need to be done in a battery rather than as a single test to ensure the greatest validity. Such noninvasive studies cannot necessarily replace an angiogram, but they are very useful as quick ways of following patients postoperatively or for those for whom operation was not felt to be suitable. They are usually done before angiography as a means of cross-checking their current accuracy in a particular patient and as a baseline for validating their future use in that patient. Coagulation tests have been of low yield. An electrocardiogram is always done and an echocardiogram rarely in patients with stroke. The former is important to show past or current disease and as a baseline for patients who will undergo surgery. The latter only rarely reveals an embolic source. The CT or MR is always done, since these studies often show evidence of silent or multiple cerebral lesions that may influence therapeutic decisions in the patient with strokes and dementia.

As mentioned, multiple cerebral infarcts are the second most common cause of dementia in the elderly. Initially the dementia was thought to be related more to the total volume of injured brain than to the locus of injury. Recently, however, small thalamic infarcts have been reported to be associated with intellectual loss (Graff-Radford, Eslinger, Demasio, et al, 1984), and so the question is still open. Hachinski, Iliff, Zilkha et al (1975) have suggested a scoring system which may be helpful in the clinical differentiation of multi-infarct dementia from Alzheimer's disease. Key items are the abruptness of onset, stepwise progression, history of stroke and the presence of focal neurologic signs and symptoms. The higher the score, the more more likely the diagnosis of multi-infarct dementia. However, many cases are not clearly delineated by this system and laboratory tests may still be required.

REFERENCES

Brown, R.G., Marsden, C.D. (1984). How common is dementia in Parkinson's disease? Lancet. 2, 1262-1265.

Cummings, J.L., Benson, D.F. (1983). Dementia. A Clinical Approach. Boston: Butterworths, 416 pp.

Folstein, M.F., Folstein, S.E., McHugh, P.R. (1975). "Mini-mental state":
A practical method for grading the cognitive state of patients for the
clinician. J. Psychiat. Res. 12, 189-198.

Graff-Radford, N.R., Eslinger, P.J., Demasio, A.R. et al. (1984).
Non-hemorrhagic infarction of the thalamus. Behavioural, anatomic &
psychologic correlates. Neurology. 34, 14-23.

Hachinski, V.C., Iliff, L.D., Zilkha, E. et al. (1975). Cerebral blood
flood and dementia. Arch. Neurol. 32, 632-637.

Hachinski, V.C., Potter, P., Mersky, H. (1987). Leuko-araiosis. Arch.
Neurol. 44, 21-23.

Katzman, R. (1986). Alzheimer's disease. NEJM. 314, 964-973.

Kokmen, E., Naessens, J.M., Offord, K.P. (1987). A short test of mental
status; description and preliminary results. Mayo Clin. Proc. 62,
281-288.

Lieberman, A., Dziatolowski, M., Kupersmith, M. et al. (1979). Dementia
in Parkinson's disease. Ann. Neurol. 6, 355-359.

Mortimer, J.A., Christensen, K.J., Webster, D. (1985). Parkinsonian
dementia. In Frederiks, J.A.M. (ed.) Handbook of Clinical Neurology,
Vol. 2(46), Neurobehavioural Disorders, Chapter 24, 371-384. Elsevier
Science Publishers B.V.

Tomlinson, B.E., Blessed, G., Roth, M. (1970). Observations on the brains
of demented old people. J. Neurol. Sci., 11, 205-242.

CHAPTER 3

NEUROPSYCHIATRIC SYNDROMES IN THE ELDERLY:

PHARMACOLOGIC MANAGEMENT

Jeffrey L. Cummings, M.D.
Veterans Administration Medical Center
UCLA School of Medicine
Los Angeles, California

The burgeoning number of elderly individuals in the population is inevitably accompanied by an increase in the number of patients with organic psychosyndromes. Degenerative disorders and vascular disease increase markedly in the aged. Similarly, trauma, some types of neoplasms, and toxic-metabolic conditions are more common in the elderly than in younger individuals. Most of these disorders are accompanied by behavioural alterations and psychopharmacologic treatment will be a major component of most therapeutic regimens. In this chapter, the prevalence of organic psychosyndromes in the elderly will be reviewed, the principal geriatric neuropsychiatric disorders will be presented, and the current approach to psychopharmacologic management of organic psychosyndromes occurring in the aged will be discussed.

PREVALENCE OF ORGANIC PSYCHOSYNDROMES IN THE ELDERLY

There have been few studies of mental illness in the elderly and even less attention has been paid to the prevalence of organic psychosyndromes in the aged group. Prevalence studies show a steady decline over the life span of affective disorders, somatization disorder, antisocial personality, schizophrenia and schizophreniform disorders, and most anxiety disorders. Severe and mild cognitive impairment, in contrast, rises dramatically in the age group over age 65 (Myers, Weissman, Tischler, Holzer, Leaf, Orvaschel, Anthony, Boyd, Burke, Kramer and Stoltzman, 1984). Among elderly men, cognitive impairment, is the most common mental disorder followed by phobia, alcohol dependence, and dysthymia. Among elderly women, cognitive impairment is the second most common psychiatric syndrome preceded by phobia and followed by dysthymia and major depressive episodes. The overall prevalence of mental disorders in those over age 65 ranges from 9 to 17 percent (Myers, Weissman, Tischler, Holzer, Leaf, Orvaschel, Anthony, Boyd, Burke, Kramer and Stoltzman, 1984; Robins, Helzer, Weissman, Orvaschel, Gruenberg, Burke and Regier, 1984). Between 1 and 9 percent of the elderly see a mental health specialist regularly, suggesting that most neuropsychiatric disorders in the aged are managed by generalists (Shapiro, Skinner, Kessler, Von Korff, German, Tischler, Leaf, Benham, Cottler and Regier, 1984).

The proportion of behavioural disorders occurring in the elderly as a product of neuromedical illness is unknown. All late-onset disorders with cognitive impairment are a result of brain dysfunction, and a considerable number of late-occurring depressions, psychoses, and personality alterations are produced by stroke, trauma, neoplasms, or toxic-metabolic disorders or are the initial manifestations of degenerative diseases. The prevalence of stroke rises exponentially from approximately 5 per 1000 at age 60 to 25 per 1000 at age 80 (Katzman, 1983). Vascular disease may present with dementia, depression, mania or psychosis as well as more elementary neurologic disorders. The prevalence of dementia of the Alzheimer type (DAT) rises from 17 per 1000 in the age group from 65 to 74 years old to 148 per 1000 in those over age 85 (Sulkava, Wikstrom, Aromaa, Raitasalo, Lehtinen, Lehtela and Palo, 1985). In the early phases, DAT may be dominated by delusions and personality alterations. Parkinson's disease, with its attendant depression and drug-induced neuropsychiatric syndromes, is infrequent under age 45 and is most prevalent between the ages of 75 and 84 years (Kurtzke and Kurland, 1983). Similarly, there is a marked increase in the number of medical illnesses in the elderly population -- up to 78 percent of patients over age 65 have four major illnesses (Wilson, Lawson and Braws, 1962) -- and secondary brain involvement may produce substantial neuropsychiatric morbidity. These observations suggest that a sizeable portion of the behavioural disorders observed in the elderly are produced by structural or metabolic brain dysfunction, and a careful search for such diseases in all older individuals with psychiatric disturbances is warranted.

Organic etiologies for behavioural abnormalities are under-recognized. Hoffman (1982) and Dubin, Weiss and Zeccardi (1983) found that idiopathic psychiatric syndromes were frequently re-diagnosed as organic mental syndromes when the patients were carefully evaluated. Koranyi (1982), in a review of several earlier studies, noted that previously undiagnosed medical illnesses were found in from 46 to 80 percent of carefully scrutinized patients with psychiatric illness and that the over-looked diseases had contributed directly to the psycho-pathology in from 9 to 46 percent of cases. Among patients with neurologic disorders, from 40 to 50 percent have psychiatric co-morbidity

(De Paulo and Folstein, 1978; Schiffer, 1983). Thus, neurologic and
systemic illnesses frequently present with psychiatric disturbances and
the differential diagnosis of behavioural alterations in the elderly
includes neurologic, medical, toxic, and primary psychiatric disorders.

OVERVIEW OF NEUROPSYCHIATRIC DISORDERS IN THE ELDERLY

Neurology has traditionally concerned itself with deficit syndromes
such as dementia, delirium, aphasia, and amnesia, whereas psychiatry has
been most involved with idiopathic behavioural disorders such as
schizophrenia, manic-depressive illness, anxiety disorders, and
personality disorders. This dichotomous approach is difficult to justify
in young patients and definitely inappropriate in the elderly. Rather,
each behavioural syndrome is approached as the possible end product of a
large number of neurologic, toxic, medical, and idiopathic psychiatric
illnesses. This applies to deficit disorders as well as "productive"
syndromes such as depression, mania, hallucinations, delusions, and
personality alterations (Cummings, 1985a). Treatment of neuropsychiatric
disorders depends on definitive etiologic diagnosis. Psychopharmacologic
management is directed at controlling the behavioural symptoms, while
simultaneous neuromedical management is applied to the underlying
disorder.

The principal neuropsychiatric syndromes requiring psychopharmacologic
management are reviewed below. These include organic affective disorders
(depressed and manic types), organic delusional disorders, organic
personality disorders, and dementia.

ORGANIC AFFECTIVE DISORDER, DEPRESSED TYPE

Table 1 lists the principal organic affective disorders and their
common neurologic, medical, and toxic etiologies.

Organic affective disorder depressed type (secondary depression,
symptomatic depression) refers to patients who have a neuromedical illness
and develop a dysphoric mood and at least two of the following: appetite
or weight change, sleep disturbance, psychomotor retardation or agitation,
anhedonia, anergia, feelings of worthlessness and self-reproach, cognitive
impairment, or suicidal ideation. Dementia, delirium, mood-incongruent
delusions, hallucinations or personality change should not dominate the
syndrome (Diagnostic and Statistical Manual of Mental Disorders [DSM-III],
1980).

TABLE 1: ORGANIC AFFECTIVE DISORDERS OF THE ELDERLY
         AND THEIR COMMON CAUSES

Neuropsychiatric Disorder	Common Neurologic Etiologies	Common Toxic and Metabolic Etiologies
Depression	Stroke Parkinson's disease Progressive supranuclear palsy Basal ganglia calcification Trauma Neoplasms CNS infections Hydrocephalus Multiple sclerosis Epilepsy	Metabolic disorders Endocrine disorders Viral infections Systemic illnesses Drugs Antihypertensive agents Sedative-hypnotics Minor tranquilizers Steroids
Mania	Huntington's disease Encephalitis Syphillis Multiple sclerosis Neoplasms Trauma Stroke	Metabolic disorders Uremia Hemodialysis Hyperthyroidism Sympathomimetics Carcinoid syndrome Vitamin B12 deficiency Drugs Levodopa Bromocriptine Sympathomimetics Iproniazid Cocaine Amphetamines Baclofen Cimetadine Metrizamide Thyroxin Corticosteroids

Etiologies

The principal neurologic conditions producing depression in the elderly include stroke, Parkinson's disease, neoplasms, trauma, central nervous system infections, epilepsy, and hydrocephalus (Cummings, 1985a; Whitlock, 1982). Robinson and colleagues (Robinson and Chait, 1985; Robinson and Price, 1982; Robinson and Szetela, 1981; Robinson, Kubos, Starr, Rao and Price, 1984; Robinson, Starr and Price, 1984) have shown that 60 percent of patients with hemispheric strokes will have a major depressive episode or symptoms of dysthymia within six months of the insult. Furthermore, the likelihood of developing depression following stroke varies with lesion location: in their studies, depression was evident among 70 percent of patients with left-sided anterior injury, 38 percent with left-posterior insults, 17 percent of those with right-posterior lesions, and none of those with right-sided anterior hemispheric lesions (Figure 1). Depression has also been reported in 60 percent of patients with multi-infarct dementia (Cummings, Miller, Hill and Neshkes, 1987).

Parkinson's disease is commonly associated with depression. Depression occasionally precedes the onset of the motor symptoms and occurs during the course of the illness in 35 to 50 percent of patients (Celesia and Wanamaker, 1972; Mayeux, Stern, Rosen and Leventhal, 1981; Santamaria, Tolosa and Valles, 1986). Depression is more severe in Parkinson's disease than in non-neurologic illnesses with equivalent motor impairment (i.e., arthritis) and is not determined by the severity of the motor disturbance. Depression is also frequent in other basal ganglia disease of the elderly including progressive supranuclear palsy, Huntington's disease, and idiopathic basal ganglia calcification.

An increased prevalence of depression has also been reported in a variety of other CNS disorders including post-traumatic encephalopathy, neoplasms, infections (Jakob-Creutzfeldt disease, chronic meningitis, acquired immune deficiency syndrome), and hydrocephalus (Cummings, 1985; Lobosky, Vangilder and Damasio, 1984; Rundell, Wise and Ursano, 1986; Whitlock, 1982). Multiple sclerosis and epilepsy, while rarely beginning in the elderly, are also associated with an increased frequency of depression (Mendez, Cummings and Benson, 1986; Schiffer, Caine, Banford and Levy, 1983; Whitlock and Siskind, 1980).

Depression occurs in up to one-third of patients with medical illness and up to one-quarter of patients with systemic illnesses experience major depressive episodes (Rodin and Voshart, 1986). Endocrine disorders (particularly hypothyroidism and Cushing's disease), viral infections, and systemic illnesses such as uremia, cardiopulmonary compromise, cancer, and hepatic encephalopathy are among the most common medical illnesses causing

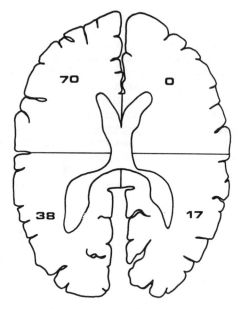

FIGURE 1: Template of the brain showing the prevalence of depression relative to lesion location in the brain (data from Robinson and Chait, 1985).

depression. Pharmaceutical agents particularly likely to induce depression include antihypertensive agents, sedative hypnotics, minor tranquillizers, and steroidal compounds (Cummings, 1985a; Lewis and Smith, 1983; Whitlock, 1982; Whitlock and Evans, 1978).

Neuromedical illnesses may produce symptoms such as motoric slowing, weight loss, and insomnia that mimic the somatic and neurovegetative manifestations of depression. Thus, the cognitive-affective symptoms such as suicidal feelings, a sense of failure, guilt, asociality, indecision, and anhedonia provide the best means of assessing depression in patients with neurologic or medical disorders (Cavanaugh, 1984; Clark, Cavanaugh and Gibbons, 1983).

Management

Medical management of secondary depressions requires evaluation and treatment of the underlying disorder as well as therapy of the mood disorder. The associated cardiovascular disease, toxic-metabolic conditions, hydrocephalus, infections or neoplasms must be evaluated and treated. Antidepressant treatment is often required in addition to management of the etiologic disorder. Table 2 presents information on psychotropic agents commonly used in the elderly. The dosages suggested in this chapter are only a *guideline for prescribing* in the elderly. In specific cases the dose required may be *above or below* these ranges. Nortriptyline and trazodone have been shown in double blind trials to be efficacious in relieving depression following stroke (Lipsey, Robinson, Pearlson, Rao and Price, 1984; Reding, Orto, Winter, Fortuna, Di Ponte and McDowell, 1986). Desipramine, nortriptyline, and imipramine have all been used successfully to treat the depression of Parkinson's disease (Anderson, Aabro, Gulmann, Hjelmsted and Pederson, 1980; Laitinen, 1969; Strang, 1965). ECT relieves depression and at least temporarily improves the motor symptoms of Parkinsonian patients (Asnis, 1977; Lebensohn and Jenkins, 1975).

Choice of antidepressant in the elderly is guided primarily by the side-effect profile of the available agents. The principal side-effects of tricyclic antidepressant agents include anticholinergic toxicity, orthostatic hypotension, and cardiotoxicity (Jenike, 1985; Salzman, 1982; Thompson, Moran and Nies, 1983). Anticholinergic effects include dry mouth, constipation, blurred vision, impotence, urinary retention, aggravation of glaucoma, and delirium. Many of these effects may potentially interact with common problems in the elderly - prostatic hypertrophy, glaucoma, presbyopia - to produce disastrous results. Amitriptyline is the most anticholinergic of the tricyclic agents followed in descending order by imipramine, doxepin, nortriptyline, and desipramine. Trazodone, a non-tricyclic agent, also has little anticholinergic activity. Orthostatic hypotension is most frequent with imipramine and least frequent with desipramine and nortriptyline. Cardiac effects of antidepressant agents include intraventricular conduction delay with prolongation of the QRS interval on EKG, decreasing cardiac return, and decreasing myocardial contractibility. An EKG should be performed prior to the initiation of tricyclic therapy and at regular intervals during continued treatment. Nortriptyline, desipramine, and trazodone appear to be the safest antidepressants available for use in elderly patients.

Monoamine oxidase inhibitors (MAOIs) (phenelzine, tranylcypromine) should be considered only when the patient has failed to respond to two traditional antidepressants. Dietary restrictions are necessary during MAOI administration, and hypertensive episodes associated with adverse drug reactions may be particularly dangerous in the elderly (Thompson, Moran and Nies, 1983). Dosage of all medications including antidepressant

TABLE 2: COMMONLY USED PSYCHOPHARMACOLOGIC AGENTS IN GERIATRIC ORGANIC AFFECTIVE DISORDERS

Class/Agent	Usual Dosage	Advantages/Disadvantages
Antidepressants		
Nortriptyline	25-50 mg/d	Little orthostatic hypotension; therapeutic window of blood level defined (50-150 ng/ml)
Desipramine	25-50 mg/d	Little anticholinergic activity
Trazodone	50-100 mg/d	Little anticholinergic activity; may cause cardiotoxicity in patients with cardiac disease
Antimanic agents		
Lithium	300-600 mg/d	Elderly patients more likely to experience adverse side effects; drug interactions common; optimal blood level is 0.4-0.7 mmol/l
Carbamazepine	600-800 mg/d	Fewer side effects than Lithium; requires monitoring of platelets and white blood cells; therapeutic level 8-12 mcg/ml

agents must be adjusted downward to allow for alterations in drug pharmacokinetics occurring in the elderly. Decreased drug metabolism and diminished availability of serum proteins to bind drugs result in an increased percentage of pharmacologically active drug in the circulation.

ORGANIC AFFECTIVE DISORDER, MANIC TYPE

Secondary mania is a rare phenomenon compared to symptomatic depression. It is manifested by an elevated, expansive, or irritable mood and at least two of the following: increase in physical or sexual activity, pressured speech, flight of ideas or racing thoughts, inflated self-esteem, decreased need for sleep, distractability, and involvement in risk-taking activities (DSM-III, 1980). An etiology should be identifiable, and dementia, delirium, delusions, and hallucinosis should not be predominant in the syndrome.

Etiologies

Secondary mania has been associated with both structural and toxic-metabolic brain disorders (Table 1). The most common neurologic disorders producing mania include Huntington's disease, encephalitis and post-encephalitic syndromes, syphilis, multiple sclerosis, neoplasms, trauma, and stroke (Cummings, 1986; Krauthammer and Klerman, 1978; Shukla, Cook, Mukherjee, Godwin and Miller, 1987). Focal lesions inducing secondary mania have usually involved the right hemisphere in the medial frontal or perithalamic regions (Cummings and Mendez, 1984).

Metabolic conditions producing mania have included uremia and hemodialysis, hyperthyroidism, pellagra, carcinoid syndrome, and vitamin B12 deficiency. Drugs that have caused manic syndromes include levodopa, bromocriptine, sympathomimetics, iproniazid, cocaine, amphetamines, baclofen, cimetidine, metrizamide, thyroxin, and corticosteroids (Cummings 1985, 1986; Krauthammer and Klerman, 1978).

Mania has been induced by a wide range of antidepressant medications including amitriptyline, imipramine, desipramine, doxepin, nortriptyline, protriptyline, MAOI, tomoxetine, trazodone, and alprazolam (Arana, Pearlman and Shader, 1985; Nasralleh, Fowler and Judd, 1982; Pickar, Murphy, Cohen, Campbell and Lipper, 1982; Steinberg and Chouinard, 1985; Warren and Bick, 1984). These patients, however, are excluded from the diagnosis of secondary mania by some definitions since they had an underlying affective disorder requiring antidepressant therapy and may have suffered from a manic-depressive disorder that was uncovered by antidepressant treatment.

Management

In addition to addressing the underlying condition, the treatment approach to patients with secondary mania includes management of the manic behaviour (Table 2). Lithium is the most widely used anti-manic agent and has been used successfully in the treatment of organic affective illness with mania (Oyewumi and Lapierre, 1981; Rosenbaum and Barry, 1975; Young, Taylor and Holmstrom, 1977). Special precautions are necessary when treating an aged individual with lithium. Lithium is excreted entirely by the kidney and reduced renal function will result in elevated lithium levels (Csernausky and Hollister, 1985; Jenike, 1985). Interactions between lithium and drugs commonly used in the elderly are also common. Thiazide diuretics decrease renal clearance and elevate serum lithium levels; and nonsteroidal anti-inflammatory drugs (indomethacin, phenylbutazone), methyldopa, and neuroleptics may lead to moderate elevations in lithium levels (Jenike, 1985; Rosenbaum, Maruta and Richelson, 1979). Lithium toxicity is evidenced by tremor, ataxia, slurred speech, and drowsiness or excitement. In a few cases, the symptoms are permanent (Donaldson and Cunningham, 1983). A serum level of 0.4 to 0.7 mmol/l is usually adequate in older patients to ameliorate manic behaviour without producing toxic manifestations.

Carbamazepine is an antimanic agent that may be used in patients unresponsive to or intolerant of lithium. Carbamazepine produces substantial improvement in 70 percent of patients within 10 days of initiating treatment. Dosages should be adjusted to produce serum levels of 8 to 12 mcg/ml (Ballenger and Post, 1980; Okuma, Inanaga, Otsuki, Sarai, Takahashi, Razama, Mori and Watanbe, 1979). There are few side effects with carbamazepine in appropriate dosages, but platelets and white blood cell counts must be followed because of the rare production of blood dyscrasias (Joffe, Post, Roy-Byrne and Unde, 1985).

ORGANIC DELUSIONAL DISORDER

Delusions are false beliefs that are firmly held despite evidence to the contrary and are not accepted by other members of the person's culture or subculture (Cummings, 1985a,b; DSM-III, 1980). Organic delusional disorder is a clinical syndrome characterized by the occurrence of prominent delusions in the setting of a neuromedical illness. Dementia, delirium, affective disturbances, or hallucinations do not dominate the syndrome (DSM-III, 1980). The diagnosis of organic delusional disorder is supported by the onset of delusions following the identification of a neuromedical illness, the absence of any history of previous psychiatric illness or premorbid personality abnormalities, and the absence of a family history of psychiatric illness (Cummings, 1985a,b, 1986). The delusions may be simple persecutory beliefs or complex, systematized constructions. They may involve misinterpretation of many aspects of one's experiences or they may be highly focused content-specific disorders such as believing that one's spouse has been replaced by an identically-appearing imposter (Capgras syndrome), concluding that one is infested (acrophobia), believing that one has a double (heutoscopy, doppelganger), or believing that one is loved by a powerful or influential figure (de Clerambault's syndrome).

Etiologies

Organic delusional disorder occurs with a wide variety of toxic-metabolic and structural brain disorders (Table 3). They are particularly common in some extrapyramidal diseases including Huntington's disease, post-encephalitic Parkinson's disease, and idiopathic basal ganglia calcification (Cummings and Benson, 1983; Cummings, 1985b). Infectious illnesses, such as herpes encephalitis, that affect the temporal lobe may present with psychosis as the initial manifestation of the illness (Drachman and Adams, 1962). Organic psychoses have also been reported following cerebrovascular insults, with cerebral neoplasms, with brain trauma, and with hydrocephalus (Cummings, 1985a; Levine and Finklestein, 1982; Nasrallah, Fowler and Judd, 1981; Trimble and Cummings, 1981). There is a well-documented tendency for patients with temporal lobe epilepsy to develop schizophrenia-like psychoses, particularly if the epileptic focus involves the left hemisphere (Perez and Trimble, 1980; Slater, Beard, Glithero, 1963). Most disturbances associated with delusions involve the limbic system or the basal ganglionic dopaminergic system.

Medical illnesses associated with organic psychoses include cardiopulmonary failure, uremia, hepatic encephalopathy, endocrine disturbances, vitamin deficiency states, and collagen vascular disorders (Cummings, 1985a,b; Freeman, 1980; McEvoy, 1981). In addition, an array of drugs have been reported to produce pyschotic experiences. Pharmacologic agents commonly used in the elderly and known to produce organic delusional disorders include anticholinergic drugs, levodopa, bromocriptine, amantadine hydrochloride, thyroxin, anticonvulsants, antidepressants, procaine penicillin, digitalis, cimetidine, metrizamide, corticosteroids, methylphenidate, amphetamines, lidocaine, procainamide, ephedrine and isoniazid (Barnhart and Bowden, 1979; Cummings 1985b; Cummings, Barritt and Horan, 1986; Davis, Cummings, Malin and Garrick, 1986; Dysken, Merry and Davis, 1978; Estroff and Gold, 1986).

TABLE 3: COMMON CAUSES OF ORGANIC DELUSIONAL
DISORDERS IN THE ELDERLY

Neurologic Disorders
    Huntington's disease
    Postencephalitic parkinsonism
    Idiopathic basal ganglia calcification
    Herpes encephalitis
    Stroke
    Trauma
    Hydrocephalus
    Epilepsy
    Neoplasms

Medical Illnesses
    Anoxia
    Uremia
    Hepatic encephalopathy
    Endocrine disorders
    Vitamin deficiency states
    Collagen-vascular disorders

Toxic Conditions
    Anticholinergic agents
    Levodopa
    Amantadine hydrochloride
    Bromocriptine
    Thyroxin
    Corticosteroids
    Anticonvulsants
    Antidepressants
    Procaine penicillin
    Digitalis
    Cimetidine
    Metrizamide
    Methylphenidate
    Amphetamines
    Lidocaine
    Procainamide
    Ephedrine
    Isoniazid

Treatment

Organic delusional syndromes may require symptomatic treatment in addition to the therapeutic interventions directed at the underlying neuromedical illness (Table 4). Neuroleptic agents are the treatment of choice for organic delusional disorders. Many antipsychotic drugs are available and selection is guided primarily by the side-effect profile of the individual agents. Low potency agents such as thioridazine have more associated orthostatic hypotension and anticholinergic side effects and may be sedating but have little tendency to produce extrapyramidal reactions. High potency drugs (i.e., haloperidol, fluphenazine hydrochloride) have fewer anticholinergic side effects, are less sedating, and have a greater risk of extrapyramidal side effects (Branchey, Lee, Amin and Simpson, 1978; Jenike, 1985; Steinhart, 1983). Elderly patients are less likely than younger patients to develop acute dystonic reactions; they are at greater risk for the development of tardive dyskinesia and drug-induced parkinsonism (Moleman, Janzen, von Bargen, Kappers, Pepplinkhuizen and Schmitz, 1986; Smith and Baldessarini, 1980; Tepper and Haas, 1979). Dosages of neuroleptic agents are markedly lower than those used for the treatment of psychoses in younger individuals (Table 4).

ORGANIC PERSONALITY SYNDROME

Organic personality syndrome is characterized by a marked change in behaviour or personality in a patient with a neuromedical illness. The syndrome has no marked dementia, delirium, hallucinosis, delusions, or affective disturbance, and the patient should manifest at least one of the following: emotional lability (i.e., explosive outbursts), poor impulse control, marked apathy and indifference, or suspiciousness (DSM-III, 1980). The change in personality is more important as a diagnostic clue to the disorder than are the specific manifestations.

Etiologies

Organic personality disorder is most often seen following head trauma where injury to the orbitofrontal regions gives rise to a "pseudo-psychopathic" behavioural syndrome (Stuss and Benson, 1986). Other disorders producing the syndrome include neoplasms, multiple strokes, epilepsy, multiple sclerosis, and thyroid or adrenal disorders. Among degenerative disorders, personality alterations may preceed cognitive deficits in Huntington's disease and Alzheimer's disease.

Anatomic correlates of personality changes have received little study, but a few clinicoanatomical correlations have been identified. Coarsened,

TABLE 4: COMMONLY USED PSYCHOPHARMACOLOGIC AGENTS
IN ELDERLY PATIENTS WITH ORGANIC DELUSIONAL
DISORDER, ORGANIC PERSONALITY DISORDER, AND
PSEUDOBULBAR PALSY

Diagnosis/Agent	Usual Dosage	Advantages/Disadvantages
ORGANIC DELUSIONAL DISORDER		
Thioridazine	50-75 mg/d	Modest anticholinergic activity; low potency; sedating
Haloperidol	2-4 mg/d	Little anticholinergic activity; risk of extrapyramidal side effects
BELLIGERENCE, RAGE		
Propranolol	40-120 mg/d	May exacerbate cardiac failure, asthma, or angina; signs of hypoglycemia blocked
PSEUDOBULBAR PALSY		
Levodopa	600 mg/d	May produce nausea, hallucinations, delusions
Amitriptyline	50 mg/d	Anticholinergic side effects common

disinhibited, and facetious behaviour is most likely to be associated with
injury to the inferior frontal lobe; apathy often follows damage to the
lateral frontal convexity; left-sided posterior hemispheric lesions are
associated with paranoia and suspiciousness; right-sided and corpus
callosum lesions may cause schizoid behaviour, and bilateral limbic system

injury produces placidity (Brooks and Mckinlay, 1983; Cummings, 1985a; Tenhouten, Hoppe, Bogen and Walter, 1986). Antisocial and borderline personality traits may be evident in adults who evidenced brain dysfunction as children, and some patients with epilepsy manifest a dogmatic overinclusive behavioural style characterized by religiosity, hypergraphia, circumstantiality, interpersonal viscosity, and hyposexuality (Andrulonis, Gluek and Stroebel, Vogel, Shapiro and Aldridge, 1980; Cummings, 1985a; Morrison and Minkoff, 1975; Quitkin and Klein, 1969; Waxman and Geschwind, 1975).

Treatment

Impulsive violent outbursts that are unprovoked or are grossly incongruent with the provocative stimulus are the major behavioural symptoms of the organic personality syndrome requiring treatment with psychopharmacologic agents. In some cases, the intermittent aggression responds to treatment with neuroleptic agents, lithium, or carbamazepine as outlined above. In addition to these drugs, propranolol hydrochoride, a beta-adrenergic blocking agent, ameliorates rage attacks and violent behaviour in a considerable number of patients (Table 4) (Elliott, 1977; Greendyke, Schuster and Wooton, 1984; Jenkins and Maruta, 1987; Ratey, Morrill and Oxenkrug, 1983; Yudofsky, Williams and Gorman, 1981). Conservative doses of Propranolol should be administered to the elderly to avoid induction of hypotension, angina, and asthma. In addition, Propranolol blocks many of the signs of hypoglycemia and should be avoided in patients receiving insulin or oral hypoglycemic agents.

The use of benzodiazepines in the treatment of aggression is controversial. Destructiveness, belligerence, and assaultiveness have often improved in patients treated with minor tranquillizers and such drugs are often useful adjuncts to neuroleptic agents in aggressive psychotic patients (Bond and Lader, 1979). In some cases, however, administration of benzodiazepines has resulted in paradoxical rage reactions and increased aggression. Patients with depression, dementia, or delirium may have their underlying condition worsened by administration of minor tranquilizers. Use of these agents should probably be restricted to those patients whose combativeness is a product of severe anxiety or in whom other more predictable treatment modalities have been exhausted. Metabolism of benzodiazepines is often markedly delayed in the elderly, leading to prolonged serum half-lives, increasing serum levels, and toxicity. Diazepam, for example, has a 20 hour serum half-life in young adults and an 80 hour half-life in 90 year olds. The pharmacokinetics of oxazepam and lorazepam change little with aging and these agents may have the greatest margin of safety in the elderly (Thompson, Moran and Nies, 1983). The usual dosage of oxazepam is 10mg three times daily and of lorazepam 0.5 to 2mg daily.

Pseudobulbar Palsy

Pseudobulbar palsy is a syndrome manifested by inappropriate mood-incongruent laughter or crying, facial weakness, dysarthria, dysphagia, exaggerated gag reflex, and increased jaw jerk. Patients are distressed by the syndrome since their affect is disproportionate or completely unrelated to their mood. The disorder is produced by bilateral corticobulbar tract lesions and is seen most commonly with cerebro-vascular disease, amyotrophic lateral sclerosis, post-traumatic encephalopathy, multiple sclerosis, and in extrapyramidal syndromes such as progressive supranuclear palsy (Cummings, 1985a).

Pseudobulbar palsy is often treatment resistant, but patients may respond to small doses of amitriptyline or levodopa (Table 4) (Schiffer, Caine, Banford and Levy, 1984; Udaka, Yamao, Nagata, Nakamura and Kameyama, 1984).

DEMENTIA

Dementia is a syndrome manifested by acquired persistent compromise in at least three of the following spheres of neuropsychological function: language, memory, visuospatial skills, personality, and abstraction-judgement (Cummings and Benson, 1983; Cummings, Benson and LoVerme, 1980). It is an etiologically nonspecific behavioural syndrome that may be reversible or irreversible. Management of dementia has two aspects: an etiologic disorder is sought and treated if therapy is available; and complicating behaviours such as delusions, depression, and agitation are treated symptomatically. Common dementia syndromes for which specific treatment is available are shown in Table 5 (Cummings and Benson, 1983). The most common dementing disorders such as DAT and Multi-infarct dementia (MID) have no specific therapy available which can restore intellectual function. Approximately 30 percent of dementias, however, may be improved by specific therapy with at least partial reversal of the intellectual deterioration (Cummings and Benson, 1983); Cummings, Benson and LoVerme, 1980; Freemon, 1976; Marsden and Harrison, 1972; Smith and Kiloh, 1981).

Delusions, depression, and agitation may be superimposed on the intellectual deficits of dementia syndromes. Rabins, Mace and Lucas, (1982) found that families of patients with irreversible dementias reported catastrophic reactions in 87 percent of patients, suspiciousness in 63 percent, delusions in 47 percent, and violence in 47 percent. Similarly, Cummings, Miller, Hill and Neshkes, (1987) found that 50 percent of patients with DAT and 50 percent with vascular dementia had delusions. Thus, delusions and violence occur in many dementia syndromes

TABLE 5: COMMON DEMENTIA SYNDROMES OF THE ELDERLY FOR WHICH SPECIFIC REMEDIAL THERAPY IS AVAILABLE

Dementia Syndrome	Treatment
Parkinson's disease	Levodopa; Bromocriptine
Depression	Antidepressant therapy
Hydrocephalus	Ventriculoperitoneal shunt
Subdural hematoma	Surgery
Neoplasm	Surgery
Chronic meningitis	Antibiotic therapy
Systemic illness	Optimize organ function
Endocrine hypofunction	Replacement therapy
Vitamin deficiency	Vitamin replacement therapy
Inflammatory disorders	Steroid therapy
Intoxication	Eliminate exposure

and may require psychopharmacologic management. The treatment approach is the same as that noted above for organic delusional and organic personality disorders.

Depression is frequent in vascular dementia and in dementia syndromes associated with extrapyramidal syndromes. Depression occurring with dementia is treated in the same way as symptomatic depression described above.

PRINCIPLES OF GERIATRIC PSYCHOPHARMOCOLOGY

Historical and examination features that should alert the clinician to the potential existence of an organic psychosyndrome include a marked change in behaviour from one's usual demeanor, onset of the behavioural alteration late in life, an absence of familial or hereditary psychiatric disturbances, an absence of premorbid personality characteristics associated with idiopathic psychiatric disturbances, the presence of clinical features atypical of idiopathic disorders, and evidence of a coexisting neuromedical illness. The management of neuropsychiatric syndromes entails therapy of the underlying etiologic process and treatment of the behavioural manifestations of the disorder.

Jenike (1985) has enunciated useful rules for appropriate psychopharmacologic treatment of geriatric age patients. Principles of therapy include: 1) diagnose prior to treatment, 2) do not avoid psychotropic agents because of the age of the patient, 3) use low doses initially and increase dosages slowly, 4) know the pharmacology of the drug prescribed, 5) monitor drug regimens and serum levels regularly, 6) avoid multiple drug therapy whenever possible, and 7) survey the patient frequently for drug side effects. Knowledge of the neuropsychiatric syndromes occurring in the elderly combined with these principles of geriatric psychopharmacology will optimize therapy of the growing number of aged patients with neuropsychiatric disorders.

ACKNOWLEDGEMENTS

This project was supported by the Veterans Administration. The manuscript was prepared by Ms. Norene Hiekel.

REFERENCES

Anderson, J., Aabro, E., Gulmann, N., Hjelmsted, A., Pedersen, H.E. (1980). Antidepressive treatment in parkinson's disease. Acta Neurol Scand., 62, 210-219.

Andrulonis, P.A., Gluek, B.C., Stroebel, C.F., Vogel, N.G., Shapiro, A.L., Aldridge, D.M. (1980). Organic brain dysfunction and the borderline syndrome. Psychiatr. Clin. North Am., 4, 47-66.

Arana, G.W., Pearlman, C., Shader, R.I. (1985). Alprazolam-induced mania: Two clinical cases. Am. J. Psychiatry, 142, 368-369.

Asnis, G. (1977). Parkinson's disease, depression, and ECT: a review and case study. Am. J. Psychiatry, 143, 195.

Ballenger, J.C., Post, R.M. (1980). Carbamazepine in manic-depressive illness: a new treatment. Am. J. Psychiatry, 137, 782-790.

Barnhart, C.C., Bowden, C.L. (1979). Toxic psychosis with cimetidine. Am. J. Psychiatry, 136, 725-726.

Bond, A., Lader, M. (1979). Benzodiazepines and aggression. In Sander, M. (ed.). Psychopharmacology of Agression. New York: Raven Press.

Branchey, M.H., Lee, J.H., Amin, R., Simpson, G.M. (1978). High-and low-potency neuroleptics in elderly psychiatric patients. JAMA, 239, 1860-1862.

Brooks, D.N., Mckinlay, W. (1983). Personality and behavioral change after severe blunt head injury - a relative's view. J. Neurol. Neurosurg. Psychiatry, 46, 336-344.

Cavanaugh, S. (1984). Diagnosing depression in the hospitalized patient with chronic medical illness. J. Clin. Psychiatry, 45, 13-16.

Celesia, G.C., Wanamaker, W.M. (1972). Psychiatric disturbances in Parkinson's disease. Dis. Nerv. Syst., 33, 577-583.

Clark, D.C., Cavanaugh, S.V., Gibbons, R.D. (1983). The core symptoms of depression in medical and psychiatric patients. J. Nerv. Ment. Dis., 171, 705-713.

Csernansky, J.G., Hollister, L.E. (1985). Using lithium in patients with cardiac and renal disease. Hosp. Form., 20, 726-735.

Cummings, J.L. (1985a). Clinical Neuropsychiatry. New York: Grune and Stratton.

Cummings, J.L. (1985b). Organic delusions: phenomenology, anatomical correlations, and review. Brit. J. Psychiatry, 146, 184-197.

Cummings, J.L. (1986). Organic psychoses. Psychiatr. Clin. North Am., 9, 293-311.

Cummings, J.L., Barritt, C.F., Horan, M. (1986). Delusions induced by procaine penicillin: case report and review of the syndrome. Int. J. Psychiatry Med., 16, 163-168.

Cummings, J.L., Benson, D.F. (1983). Dementia: A Clinical Approach. Boston: Butterworths.

Cummings, J.L., Benson, D.F., LoVerme, S. Jr. (1980). Reversible dementia. JAMA, 243, 2434-2439.

Cummings, J.L., Gosenfeld, L.F., Houlihan, J.P., McCaffrey T. (1983). Neuropsychiatric disturbances associated with idiopathic calcification of the basal ganglia. Biol. Psychiatry, 18, 591-601.

Cummings, J.L., Mendez, M.F. (1984). Secondary mania with focal cerebrovascular lesions. Am. J. Psychiatry, 141, 1084-1087.

Cummings, J.L., Miller, B., Hill, M.A., Neshkes, R. (1987). Neuropsychiatric aspects of multi-infarct dementia and dementia of the alzheimer type. Arch. Neurol., 44, 389-393.

Davis, R.J., Cummings, J.L., Malin, B.D., Garrick, T. (1986). Prolonged psychosis with first-rank symptoms following metrizamide myelography. Psychosomatics, 27, 373-375.

DePaulo, J.R. Jr, Folstein, M.F. (1978). Psychiatric disturbances in neurological patients: detection, recognition, and hospital course. Ann. Neurol., 4, 225-228.

Diagnostic and statistical manual of mental disorders. American Psychiatric Association, Washington, D.C., 1980.

Donaldson, I. MacG., Cunningham, J. (1983). Persisting neurologic sequelae of Lithium Carbonate therapy. Arch. Neurol., 40, 747-751.

Drachman, D.A., Adam, R.D. (1962). Herpes simplex and acute inclusion-body encephalitis. Arch. Neurol., 7, 561-566.

Dubin, W.R., Weiss, K.T., Zeccardi, J.A. (1983). Organic brain syndrome. The psychiatric imposter. JAMA, 249, 60-62.

Dysken, M.W., Merry, W., Davis, J.M. (1978). Anticholinergic psychoses. Psychiatry Ann., 8, 452-456.

Elliott, F.A. (1977). Propranolol for the control of belligerent behaviour following acute brain damage. Ann. Neurol., 1, 489-491.

Estroff, T.W., Gold, M.S. (1986). Medication-induced and toxin-induced psychiatric disorders. In Extein, I., Gold, M.S. (ed.). Medical Mimics of Psychiatric Disorders. Washington, D.C.: American Psychiatric Press, 163-198.

Freeman, A.M. III. (1980). Delusion, depersonalization, and unusual psychopathological symptoms. In Hall, R.C.W. (ed.). Psychiatric Presentations of Medical Illness. New York: SP Medical & Scientific Books, 75-89.

Freemon, F.R. (1976). Evaluation of patients with progressive intellectual deterioration. Arch. Neurol. 33, 658-659.

Greendyke, R.M., Schuster, D.B., Wooton, J.A. (1984). Propranol in the treatment of assaultive behavior with organic brain disease. J. Clin. Psychopharmacol., 4, 282-285.

Hoffman, R.S. (1982). Diagnostic errors in the evaluation of behavioural disorders. JAMA, 248, 964-967.

Jenike, M.A. (1985). Handbook of Geriatric Psycho-pharmacology. Littleton, Massachusetts: PSG Publishing Company.

Jenkins, S.C., Maruta, T. (1987). Therapeutic use of propranolol for intermittent explosive disorder. Mayo Clin. Proc., 62, 204-214.

Joffe, R.T., Post. R.M., Roy-Byrne, P.P., Unde, T.W. (1985). Hematological effects of carbamazepine in patients with affective illness. Am. J. Psychiatry, 142, 1196-1199.

Katzman, R. (1983). Demography, definitions and problems. In Katzman, R., Terry, R. (eds.). The Neurology of Aging. Philadelphia: F.A. Davis Company, 1-14.

Koranyi, E.K. (1982). Undiagnosed physical illness in psychiatric patients. Annu. Rev. Med., 33, 309-316.

Krauthammer, C., Klerman, G.L. (1978). Secondary mania. Arch. Gen. Psychiatry, 35, 1333-1339.

Kurtzke, J.F., Kurland, L.T. (1983). The epidemiology of neurologic disease. In Baker, A.B., Joynt, R.J. (eds.). Clinical Neurology. New York: Harper and Row, 1-143.

Laitinen. L. (1969). Desipramine in treatment of Parkinson's disease. Acta. Neurol. Scand., 45, 109-113.

Lebensohn, Z.M., Jenkins, R.B. (1975). Improvement of parkinsonism in depressed patients treated with ECT. Am. J. Psychiatry, 131, 83-285.

Levine, D.N., Finklestein, S. (1982). Delayed psychosis after right temporoparietel stroke or trauma: relation to epilepsy. Neurology, 32, 267-273.

Lewis, D.A., Smith, R.E. (1983). Steroid-induced psychiatric syndromes. J. Affect. Dis., 5, 319-332.

Lipsey, D.R., Robinson, R.G., Pearlson, G.D., Rao, K., Price, T.R. (1984). Nortriptyline treatment of post-stroke depression: a double-blind study. Lancet, 1, 297-300.

Lobosky, J.M., Vangilder, J.C., Damasio, A.R. (1984). Behavioural manifestations of third ventricular colloid cysts. J. Neurol. Neurosurg. Psychiatry, 47, 1075-1080.

Marsden, C.D., Harrison, M.J.G. (1972). Outcome of investigation of patients with presenile dementia. Brit. Med. J. 2, 249-252.

Mayeux, R., Stern, Y., Rosen, J., Leventhal, J. (1981). Depression, intellectual impairment, and parkinson's disease. Neurology, 31, 645-650.

McEvoy, J.P. (1981). Organic brain syndromes. Ann. Intern. Med., 95, 212-220.

Mendez, M.F., Cummings, J.L., Benson, D.F. (1986). Depression in epilepsy. Arch. Neurol., 43, 766-770.

Moleman, P., Janzen, G., von Bargen, B.A., Kappers, E.J., Pepplinkhuizen, L., Schmitz, P.I.M. (1986). Relationship between age and incidence of parkinsonism in psychiatric patients treated with haloperidol. Am. J. Psychiatry, 143, 232-234.

Morrison, J.R., Minkoff, K. (1975). Explosive personality as a sequel to the hyperactive-child syndrome. Compr. Psychiatry, 16, 343-348.

Myers, J.K., Weissman, M.M., Tischler, G.L., Holzer, C.E. III, Leaf, P.J., Orvaschel, H., Anthony, J.C., Boyd, J.H., Burke, J.F. Jr, Kramer, M., Stoltzman, R. (1984). Six-month prevalence of psychiatric disorders in three communities. Arch. Gen. Psychiatry, 1, 959-967.

Nasrallah, H.A., Fowler, R.C., Judd, L.L. (1982). Schizophrenia-like illness following head injury. Psychosomatics, 22, 359-361.

Nasrallah, H.A., Lyskowski, J., Schroeder, D. (1982). TCA-induced mania: differences between switchers and nonswitchers. Biol. Psychiatry, 17, 271-274.

Okuma, T., Inanaga, K., Otsuki, S., Sarai, K., Takahashi, R., Razama, H., Mori, A., Watanabe, M. (1979). Comparison of the antimanic efficacy of carbamazepine and chlorpromazine: a double-blind controlled study. Psychopharmacology, 66, 211-217.

Oyewumi, L.K., Lapierre, Y.D. (1981). Efficacy of lithium in treating mood disorders occurring after brain stem injury. Am. J. Psychiatry, 138, 110-112.

Perez, M.M., Trimble, M.R. (1980). Epileptic psychosis - diagnostic comparison with process schizophrenia. Brit. J. Psychiatry, 137, 245-249.

Pickar, D., Murphy, D.L., Cohen, R.M., Campbell, I.C., Lipper, S. (1982). Selective and nonselective monoamine oxidase inhibitors. Arch. Gen. Psychiatry, 39, 535-540.

Quitkin, F., Klein, D.F. (1969). Two behavioural syndromes in young adults related to possible minimal brain dysfunction. J. Psychiatry Res., 7, 131-142.

Rabins, P.V., Mace, N.L., Lucas, M.J. (1982). The impact of dementia on the family. JAMA, 248, 333-335.

Ratey, J.J., Morrill, R., Oxenkrug, G. (1983). Use of Propranolol for provoked and unprovoked episodes of rage. Am. J. Psychiatry, 140, 1356-1357.

Reding, M.J., Orto, L.A., Winter, S.W., Fortuna, I.M., Di Ponte, P., McDowell, F.H. (1986). Antidepressant therapy after stroke. Arch. Neurol., 43, 763-765.

Robins, L.N., Helzer, J.E., Weissman, M.M., Orvaschel, H., Gruenberg, E., Burke, J.D. Jr, Regier, D.A. (1984). Lifetime prevalence of specific psychiatric disorders in three sites. Arch. Gen. Psychiatry, 41, 949-958.

Robinson, R.G., Chait, T.M. (1985). Emotional correlates of structural brain injury with particular emphasis on post-stroke mood disorders. Crit. Rev. Clin. Neurobiol., 1, 285-318.

Robinson, R.G., Kubos, K.L., Starr, L.B., Rao, K., Price, T.R. (1984). Mood disorders in stroke patients. Brain, 107, 81-93.

Robinson, R.G., Price, T.R. (1982). Post-stroke depressive disorders: a follow-up study of 103 patients. Stroke, 13, 635-641.

Robinson, R.G., Starr, L.B., Price, T.R. (1984). A two year longitudinal study of mood disorders following stroke. Brit. J. Psychiatry, 144, 256-262.

Robinson, R.G., Szetela, B. (1981). Mood change following left hemispheric brain injury. Ann. Neurol., 9, 447-453.

Rodin, G., Voshart, K. (1986). Depression in the medically ill: an overview. Am. J. Psychiatry, 143, 696-705.

Rosenbaum, A.H., Barry, M.J. Jr. (1975). Positive therapeutic response to lithium in hypomania secondary to organic brain syndrome. Am. J. Psychiatry, 132, 1072-1073.

Rosenbaum, A.H., Maruta, T., Richelson, E. (1979). Drugs that alter mood. Lithium. Mayo Clin. Proc., 54, 401-407.

Rundell, J.R., Wise, M.G., Ursano, R.J. (1986). Three cases of AIDS-related psychiatric disorders. Am. J. Psychiatry, 143, 777-778.

Salzman, C. (1982). A primer on geriatric psychopharmacology. Am. J. Psychiatry, 139, 67-74.

Santamaria, J., Tolosa, E., Valles, A. (1986). Parkinson's disease with depression: a possible subgroup of idiopathic parkinsonism. Neurology, 36, 1130-1133.

Schiffer, R.B. (1983). Psychiatric aspects of clinical neurology. Am. J. Psychiatry, 140, 205-207.

Schiffer, R.B., Caine, E.D., Banford, K.A., Levy, S. (1983). Depressive episodes in patients with multiple sclerosis. Am. J. Psychiatry, 140, 1498-1500.

Schiffer, R.B., Herndon, R.M., Rudick, R.A. (1985). Treatment of pathologic laughing and weeping with amitriptyline. N. Engl. J. Med., 312, 1480-1482.

Shapiro, S., Skinner, E.A., Kessler, L.G., Von Korff, M., German, P.S., Tischler, G.L., Leaf, P.J., Benham, L., Cottler, L., Regier, D.A.

(1984). Utilization of health and mental health services. Arch. Gen. Psychiatry, 41, 971-978.

Shukla, S., Cook, B.L., Mukherjee, S., Godwin, C., Miller, M.G. (1987). Mania following head trauma. Am. J. Psychiatry, 144, 93-96.

Slater, E., Beard, A.W., Glithero, E. (1963). The schizophrenia-like psychoses of epilepsy. Brit. J. Psychiatry, 109, 95-150.

Smith, J.M., Baldessarini, R.J. (1980). Changes in prevalence, severity, and recovery in tardive dyskinesia with age. Arch. Gen. Psychiatry, 37, 1368-1373.

Smith, J.S., Kiloh, L.G. (1981). The investigation of dementia: results in 200 consecutive admissions. Lancet, 1, 824-827

Steinberg, S., Chouinard, G. (1985). A case of mania associated with tomoxetine. Am. J. Psychiatry, 142, 1517-1518.

Steinhart, M.J. (1983). The use of haloperidol in geriatric patients with organic mental disorder. Curr. Ther. Res., 33, 132-143.

Strang, R.R. (1965). Imipramine in treatment of parkinsonism: a double-blind placebo study. Brit. Med. J., 2, 33-34.

Stuss, D.T., Benson, D.F. (1986). The Frontal Lobes. New York: Raven Press.

Sulkava, R., Wikstrom, J., Aromaa, A., Raitasalo, R., Lehtinen, V., Lehtela, K., Palo, J. (1985). Prevalence of severe dementia in Finland. Neurology, 35, 1025-1029.

Tenhouten, W.D., Hoppe, K.D., Bogen, JE., Walter, D.O. (1986). Alexithymia: an experimental study of cerebral commissurotomy patients and normal control subjects. Am. J. Psychiatry, 143, 312-316.

Tepper, S.J., Haas, J.F. (1979). Prevalence of tardive dyskinesia. J. Clin. Psychiatry, 40, 508-516.

Thompson, J.L. II, Moran, M.G., Nies, A.S. (1983). Psychotropic drug use in the elderly. N. Engl. J. Med. 308, 134-138, 194-199.

Trimble, M.R., Cummings, J.L. (1981). Neuropsychiatric disturbances following brainstem lesions. Brit. J. Psychiatry, 138, 56-59.

Udaka, F., Yamao, S., Nagata, H., Nakamura, S., Kameyama, M. (1984) Pathologic laughing and crying treated with levodopa. Arch. Neurol., 41, 1095-1096.

Warren, M., Bick, P.A. (1984). Two case reports of trazodone-induced mania. Am. J. Psychiatry, 141, 1103-1104.

Waxman, S.G., Geschwind, N. (1975). The interictal behaviour syndrome of temporal lobe epilepsy. Arch. Gen. Psychiatry, 32, 1580-1586.

Whitlock, F.A. (1982). Symptomatic Affective Disorders. New York: Academic Press.

Whitlock, F.A., Evans, L.E.J. (1978). Drugs and depression. Drugs, 15, 53-71.

Whitlock, F.A., Siskind, M.M. (1980). Depression as a major symptom of multiple sclerosis. J. Neurol. Neurosurg. Psychiatry, 43, 861-865.

Wilson, L.A., Lawson, I.R., Braws, W. (1962). Multiple disorders in the elderly. A clinical and statistical study. Lancet, 2, 841-847.

Young, L.D., Taylor, I., Holmstrom, V. (1977). Lithium treatment of patients with affective illness associated with organic brain symptoms. Am. J. Psychiatry, 134, 1405-1407.

Yudofsky, S., Williams, D., Gorman, J. (1981). Propranolol in the treatment of rage and violent behaviour in patients with chronic brain syndromes. Am. J. Psychiatry, 138, 218-220.

CHAPTER 4

PSYCHODYNAMIC PERSPECTIVES IN THE CLINICAL

APPROACH TO BRAIN DISEASE IN THE ELDERLY

Gene D. Cohen, M.D., Ph.D.
National Institute of Mental Health
Rockville, Maryland

Psychodynamic considerations in the clinical approach to brain disease in the elderly have been poorly understood and significantly overlooked, although many opportunities for clinical intervention are based upon psychodynamic factors in these disorders. Psychodynamics has been defined as the "science of mental forces and motivations that influence human behaviour and mental activity. The role of unconscious motivation in the causation of human behaviour is emphasized" (Gelfand, 1980, p. 3350). With a brain-diseased older patient, psychodynamic concerns relate to the interaction with significant others, the manifestation of symptoms and the response to treatment.

The degree of cognitive impairment or stage of illness varies considerably in brain disease in the elderly. In the early stage of Alzheimer's disease, the patient retains a high degree of cognitive awareness and hence, a sensitivity to psychodynamic turmoil. Even at an advanced stage of dementia, however, psychodynamic considerations arise, particularly in the interactions between patient and caregiver. Psychodynamic phenomena in the latter commonly have a major influence on the clinical management of the former (Cohen, 1985).

Psychodynamics should not be confused with being synonymous with psychoanalysis. Psychoanalysis as a treatment approach, is but one form of numerous intervention strategies that benefit from psychodynamic considerations. While most would consider psychoanalysis neither indicated nor practical in brain-diseased older patients, regardless of their stage of illness, psychodynamic perspectives can aid treatment planning aimed at alleviating symptoms and maximizing coping.

Dementing disorders in general, and Alzheimer's disease in particular, are marked by their degree of behavioural symptomatology. In its statement on the "Differential Diagnosis of Dementing Diseases", the National Institutes of Health Consensus Development Conference pointed out that "dementia is primarily a behavioural diagnosis". (U.S. Department of Health and Human Services, 1987), thereby separating etiologic considerations from clinical manifestations. The absence of characteristic somatic symptoms and laboratory findings is, of course, what makes the diagnosis of Alzheimer's disease so difficult, but the nature of the behavioural and psychosocial problems defines treatment opportunities (Group for the Advancement of Psychiatry, 1988; Cohen, 1984; Teri, Larson, and Reifler, 1988; Merriam, Aronson, Gaston, Wey, and Katz, 1988; Reifler and Larson, 1988). While the influence of pathophysiologic brain changes on behaviour is becoming better understood, the role of psychodynamics in the same patients has become blurred. Research needs to advance along both axes on the interaction of the two factors.

BRIEF REVIEW OF THE LITERATURE

The literature relating to psychodynamics in brain diseased older patients is not new, and it is sparse (Group for the Advancement of Psychiatry, 1988; Brink, 1979; Steury and Blank, 1977). Hollos and Ferenczi (1925), for example, wrote a book on Psychoanalysis and the Psychic Disorder of General Paresis, while Grotjahn (1940) described his psychoanalytic investigation of a 71 year old man with senile dementia (seen daily for five months).

Goldfarb (1953; 1954), in particular, heightened awareness of psychodynamics in the clinical manifestations and symtomatic responsiveness of older patients with organic mental disorders -- particularly those in the nursing home setting. He described the fear and rage experienced by these patients in response to decreased mastery, and conversely, their increased comfort following the therapist's tactful use of transference techniques that accommodated greater dependency needs.

Verwoerdt (1981) discussed possible links between premorbid personality traits and the development of certain symptoms in senile dementia. He described "compulsive, rigid individuals" as being "prone to react with profound anxiety when faced with the necessity of changing their habitual style and accommodating themselves to ego-alien constraints" (p. 189). Additionally, Verwoerdt discussed changes in autonomous ego functions (eg., greater frequency of primary process thinking), types of defenses selected (eg. increased denial and regression), and transference phenomena (eg., hostile responses).

Dream content, too, has been examined in association with organic impairment (Altschuler, Barad, and Goldfarb, 1963; Nathan, Rose-Itkoff, and Lord, 1981). Nathan et al found an increase in "loss" content in the dreams of older patients with brain atrophy.

PRACTICAL PSYCHODYNAMICS

One is often tempted to assume that, if symptoms are due to brain changes then one is dealing with biology and not psychodynamics, as if neither a healthy nor a diseased brain, per se, has anything to do with psychodynamic phenomena, and as if biological and psychosocial factors never interact. To the extent that one fails to take the opportunity to explore psychodynamic contributions to symptom manifestation in brain diseased older patients, an incomplete, if not ineffective treatment plan will often result. The series of case examples to follow will help to illustrate some, among the many different, ways that psychodynamic phenomena influence symptom formation and treatment response in such patients.

Excess Disability

Mr. K, a 72-year-old retired engineer, presented with a 15-month history of slowly worsening concentration, memory impairment, performance errors in paperwork, agitated depression, sleep disturbance, and a progressive weight loss of 40 pounds. Following comprehensive general medical, neurological and psychiatric evaluations, the clinical impression was early Alzheimer's disease with depression.

Further history of note was the patient's longstanding pattern of "overreacting" (as his wife described it), whenever he felt less in control of a situation, and, especially, if he felt he had a health problem. His wife also described her husband as being rather dependent upon her. Apparent, too, from the interview with Mrs. K, was her high degree of anxiety which unconsciously may have been compounding her husband's experience of an expanding loss of control of both his internal and external environments.

Individual psychotherapy was initiated with Mr. K, combined with consultation to Mrs. K and joint sessions with both of them. Within a week, Mr. K's mood began to improve. For the first time in over a year he began to gain weight, and reported less difficulty with concentration. These changes were paralleled by a marked reduction of Mrs. K's anxiety.

Antidepressant medication was added three weeks later which was followed by a gradual improvement in Mr. K's sleep pattern. The medication also appeared to have a positive psychological effect on the patient, seeming to provide him with a more secure sense that actions were being taken to restore order. His concentration continued to improve over the next three months and remained stable for the next year and a half, and while performance errors continued they were reported to be fewer in number. It was not until three years later that Mr. K's overall intellectual performance declined in comparison to that of the initial visit. Mood and weight, though, were still stable.

This case example illustrates several points. Foremost is the classical demonstration of the phenomenon of excess disability in Alzheimer's disease. The concomitance depression compounded the magnitude of impairment caused by Mr. K's dementia leading to excess disability. When the depression lifted, he actually clinically improved at that point in time, despite the fact that the underlying pathophysiology was that of a progressive brain disease. Excess disability is common in dementia patients, as is the ability to modify it through appropriate interventions (Reifler and Larson, 1988).

A definitive explanation of the cause of depression in Alzheimer's disease remains a research question, but there is evidence to point to both endogenous (biological) and nonendogenous (psychosocial) factors. Biological explanations address the neural degeneration that occurs in the nucleus locus ceruleus in the brains of Alzheimer victims (Bondareff, Mountjoy, Roth, Rosser, Iversen, Reynolds and Hauser, 1987). The locus ceruleus is rich in norepinephrine-producing neurons, norepinephrine being a neurotransmitter found to be diminished in neurochemical studies of depression in general. But is also may be hypothesized that psychosocial factors can induce depression in Alzheimer's disease -- particularly in the early to middle stages of the disorder, when patients (like Mr. K) can observe their own decline. Certainly, Mr. K's history of longstanding dependency problems and vulnerability to stress when his obsessive-compulsive defenses do not protect him adequately, suggest psychodynamic influences on his excess disability, as does his positive therapeutic response to individual psychotherapy and family therapy, prior to the use of antidepressant medication.

The prevalence of depression in Alzheimer patients, as well as in their close, caregiving relatives, is high, although treatment response is good. One study found that 31% of 131 Alzheimer patients were depressed. With treatment, 85% showed improvement in mood, activities of daily living, and vegetative signs (e.g. sleep, appetite and weight) (Reifler, Larson, Teri and Poulson, 1986). Family studies have reported that 25% to

81% of spousal caregivers of Alzheimer patients develop clinically significant symptoms of depression during the course of the disorder (Gallagher, 1987).

The Significance of the Patient's History

The admonition about not overlooking psychodynamics in the face of prominent brain changes in the elderly can, in part, be addressed through careful attention to the patient's history. A carefully taken history, aided by family input, is the best way to find clues of psychodynamic phenomena which might be affecting the nature and magnitude of symptoms, as well as the response to treatment. In the case which follows, an aspect of the patient's premorbid personality persisted during the course of her dementia and facilitated an important intervention strategy.

Mrs. A., an 80-year-old widow, was seen at the request of her family who indicated that they were considering placement in a nursing home. Mrs. A. lived alone in an independent-living apartment building for older adults. She had a son and a daughter who regularly called her to see how she was doing, and dropped by, as necessary, to assist with grocery shopping and related needs. Over the preceding couple of years she had been experiencing worsening memory difficulties, and, more latterly, had begun to wander from her apartment, particularly in the evening. It was her wandering that especially worried her family and neighbours, who feared that she would get lost or be harmed. They felt that, because of her wandering, Mrs. A. no longer would be able to live by herself in her apartment.

A comprehensive evaluation produced results which were consistent with a diagnosis of Alzheimer's disease. Consultation with the family proved very interesting, and revealed an intriguing theme. More with fondness than with a patronizing tone, the patient's son and daughter described their mother as having gone through life as a good "sheep", always following the recommendations of responsible authority figures, and especially doctors. Thinking about this characterization of her personality, I wondered whether, if Mrs. A. was so responsive to authoritative instructions, she might follow such advice written out on a large note to be attached to the inside of her door. I recommended that we tape a large prescription onto her apartment door that would read, "please do not leave your apartment after 5:00 p.m. in the evening." It was with some amusement and skepticism that the family participated in this effort, but to the awe of all, this strategy had a major impact on Mrs. A.'s wandering. Conferring with the neighbours during the first few weeks after placing the note on her door, we learned that her wandering had diminished noticeably, and the general concern about Mrs. A.'s safety had greatly abated.

The patient was then advised that a series of additional steps also needed to be taken. Again, she was quite compliant. Some housekeeping assistance was arranged, not only to help with chores around the apartment, but also to provide more structure to Mrs. A.'s daily routine. At first she was hesitant about having a stranger come into her apartment, but with my strong assurance, which continued in supportive, follow-up visits, she acquiesced. In addition, most of her medications were rearranged so as to be taken once or twice a day. This change allowed the son and daughter to develop a system whereby one of them called each morning and evening to remind their mother to take her medicine, remaining on the phone until she did so.

In this manner, memory patches were devised that were sufficiently effective that Mrs. A. was able to remain in her apartment (to which she was very attached) for another two years. At that point, it became apparent that she needed to be in a more protected environment. Her response to these interventions appeared to have been aided by certain psychodynamic tendencies in her personality structure.

Catastrophic Reactions

With the decline in intellectual functioning and skills that accompany dementias, patients' frustration levels also drop. These individuals commonly react with marked agitation and confusion, to stress such as difficulty with a given task, or failure. The term "catastrophic reaction" (Goldstein, 1942) refers to this phenomenon of overreacting or being excessively anxious when confronted with everyday challenges, even minor ones, such as remembering a phone number or buttoning a shirt (Mace and Rabins, 1981). It is, of course, normal, in the absence of dementia, to become frustrated when experiencing ongoing difficulties in confronting a series of challenges. One sees this, as well, with small children, who may throw temper tantrums when frustrated by a lack of gratification. In the latter instance one may understand the psychodynamics of the child's anxiety as a response to a lack of mastery. With adults as well as children, a recommended intervention is to periodically take a break from a challenging task or to seek a diversion - in more psychodynamic terms, to employ defensive maneuvers of distancing or distraction, which are often quite effective with the young child who is in a tirade.

Unfortunately, such psychodynamic lessons are too often forgotten in dealing with catastrophic reactions in Alzheimer's disease and related brain diseases in older adults. Medications are frequently substituted for psychodynamically oriented intervention which could well be faster and more effective, as well as safer. This is especially so in that catastrophic

reactions, though stormy, are typically brief. Consider the following
case example.

> Mrs. S., a 76-year-old woman with dementia, would frequently approach
> staff, visitors, and other residents on her unit at the nursing home,
> talking in an agitated manner about her deceased husband as if he were
> alive. Those who knew he had died were often uncomfortable during
> this interaction, unsure of how to respond. Some tried to explain to
> Mrs. S. that her husband was no longer living, but this often provoked
> further agitation in her.
>
> During one of my consultations to the home, the staff presented her
> case to me. I suggested that, rather than confronting Mrs. S. with
> the unreality of her thinking, a gentle distraction designed to shift
> her conversation onto another topic - one based upon reality - might
> prove more comforting to her. Learning that she had three children, I
> recommended that the next time Mrs. S. engaged a staff member about
> her husband, the person say to her something to the effect of, "I
> understand that you also have three children; can you tell me about
> them?" Interestingly, just as we were all leaving the conference room,
> Mrs. S. appeared and came up to me, of all people, and started to ask
> me when her husband was coming to visit. A dramatic hush descended,
> and all ears were in my direction. I used the line I had suggested,
> and to her relief and mine, she responded very well, moving the
> discussion onto items about her children.

Mrs. S.'s confusion about her husband caused anxiety in the patient.
Confronting this confusion directly only compounded it, adding to the
anxiety. Psychodynamically, the mental maneuver that was indicated was
not confrontation, but distraction in the direction of a reality-based,
alternative area of cognitive focus.

PSYCHODYNAMICS AND ADVANCED DEMENTIA

Referring back to the definition of psychodynamics, it should be noted
that while mental forces and motivations influence behaviour, perceptions
also play a part. Perceptions both influence and are influenced by mental
forces; this is apparent in transference reactions. Moreover, psychodynamic phenomena need to be looked at not just as internal forces
affecting the inner experience and surface symptomatology of the patient,
but as interactive dynamics affecting the relationship of the patient with
significant others. Here, too, perceptions are important -- perceptions
on the part of significant others, as much as the patient (Brody, 1986).
Such applies even at an advanced stage of dementia, when a psychodynamic

sensitivity to patient/caregiver interactions can expand one's understanding of a problem situation and one's ideas of how to intervene. The following is a case in point.

> Mrs. M. was a 97-year-old widow, mother of one daughter and two sons, who had been in a nursing home for nearly a year. One of her sons, who lived about 500 miles away, requested a psychiatric re-evaluation of Mrs. M. He was quite distraught about the family "coming apart" because of his mother's placement in the nursing home. He described a scenario in which his sister lived near the nursing home and with whom his mother had lived before needing to be institutionalized. She regularly visited her mother but was very upset at the end of each visit because of her mother's invariable question, "when am I going home?" A second brother also lived in the vicinity of the nursing home. When he visited his mother, their get-togethers ended the same way, with the same question. He became so overwhelmed by guilt feelings about "leaving" his mother in the nursing home, that he felt no longer able to face her, and stopped visiting her.

> The sister, also struggling with intense guilt feelings, became increasingly resentful about having most of the responsibility for visiting fall on her shoulders alone. Verbal fights developed among the siblings, and a growing emotional distance. Moreover, doubts ensued as to whether the correct decision had been made about Mrs. M. going to the nursing home in the first place. The family began to wonder if the diagnosis of progressive dementia was accurate. They also started to worry that their mother's expressed desire to go home reflected maltreatment by the nursing home staff. This latter fear had led the sister to become very impatient with the nursing home staff, resulting in mounting accusations and angry interactions. It was in this context that the brother who lived out-of-state asked that his mother be examined to see if her diagnosis was correct. He wanted an assessment of whether she was receiving appropriate care and hoped for some advice on how to calm the family storm.

> After acquiring background information on the patient from the family and available medical records, I went to the nursing home, reviewed the chart, and then attempted to observe the patient from a distance prior to conducting a face-to-face evaluation. Ideally, observations from a distance work out best when the patient is in the day room, having some interaction with other residents on the unit, or simply walking or sitting in some open space on the unit. The purpose of observing patients in this manner is to get a general sense of how they seem to be adjusting to their environment. Do they look comfortable or agitated; how compatible with them do their surroundings appear to be?

In observing Mrs. M. as she slowly moved about the day room with the aid of a walker, she seemed to be reasonably at ease. The most curious thing about her activity was her tendency to periodically rearrange some of the light furniture in the day room. This went on intermittently for more than 15 minutes before she stopped to rest, sat down, and fell asleep briefly, in her chair. She then got up and started to walk slowly around the unit, again with no apparent distress. At this point, I went to introduce myself to her and escorted her to her room to conduct a direct evaluation. It quickly became apparent that her capacity to give any history or organized information was extremely limited. Her cognitive impairment was such that she could not count backwards from 10, nor did she know her middle or last names.

The diagnostic work-up that previously had been carried out on her, together with the assessment that I performed, seemed to point strongly to an advanced stage of Alzheimer's disease. It appeared, too, that her dementia had been nearly this severe at the time of her admission; this, coupled with the fact that she had become incontinent around the clock at home, led the family to explore nursing home arrangements. Rather than the question being whether or not she should be in the nursing home, I wondered how the family was able to manage her at home as long as they did. Moreover, the daughter who was caring for her at home was 70 years old herself -- reflecting that late 20th century phenomenon of the 4-generation family, where the children caring for their aging parents often are themselves, senior citizens.

I returned to the nursing station to discuss the patient in more detail with the staff. While we were talking, Mrs. M. came out of her room and gradually made her way to the day room. Once there, she again started to move the furniture around. I turned to one of the nurses and asked her how often Mrs. M. moved the furniture. The nurse indicated that this was a daily event. Once, when she had asked Mrs. M. why she was doing that, the patient responded, with a sense of righteous indignation, "this is my living room; I'll move my furniture if I want to!". The nurse went on to explain that the family had told her that Mrs. M. had always taken extreme pride in the appearance of her apartment before she developed Alzheimer's disease, and that she had been a very content homebody. A certain logic occurred to me, that if Mrs. M. so frequently felt that she was in her living room, then she could not, as the family feared, constantly be dwelling on going home, since, in her mind, she was home straightening out her furniture. I wondered if her family knew that Mrs. M. experienced the day room in this manner, since they, too, might then realize their mother was more at peace with the nursing home than they recognized.

In fact, the family did not know about their mother's perception of
the day room, and upon hearing about it were surprised and somewhat
relieved. I explained further that her diagnosis was correct, that I
felt the nursing home placement was entirely appropriate and
unavoidable - if not overdue at the time of her admission - and that
she was, on the whole, making a reasonable adjustment and receiving
responsible care. In response, the family's overall level of distress
began to drop noticeably. A tremendous burden of guilt was partially
removed from their shoulders.

I suggested further that Mrs. M.'s voicing of "when am I going home"
may have taken on ritualistic or symbolic significance, and not have a
literal meaning. Instead of wondering when she was going home,
perhaps she was wondering when they would be getting together again.
Often the Alzheimer patient uses substitute words for the one
intended. Mrs. M. may have been using a substitute phrase. I
recommended to the family, that when Mrs. M. expressed her question
about going home, they might respond in at least two ways. First,
they might say something to the effect that, "Mom, you have had
different homes during your life; you are in one of your homes now."
Then, they might say, "and Mom, if you are wondering when we will be
back to see you, it will be soon." The family felt relieved by my
assessment of their mother's situation, and comfortable with the
recommended responses.

On subsequent follow-up, I learned that the tension in the family had
greatly eased, with communication among the siblings restored. The
brother, who lived near the nursing home, resumed his visits, rapport
with the nursing staff improved, and Mrs. M. continued moving her
furniture.

Though Mrs. M. had significant cognitive impairment, with limited
ability to communicate ideas and feelings, a psychodynamic assessment
nonetheless helped to alleviate the crisis that had developed. By
looking behind the superficial behaviour a new perspective on the
potential meaning of her actions was developed. This understanding,
when conveyed to the family, helped to alter their perception of the
situation. In the process, affect, behaviour, and interactions within
the family system as a whole benefited.

Biography Versus Biology

As emphasized above, the patient's history is clearly the essential
doorway allowing access to a psychodynamic understanding of the
individual. The history also has psychodynamic significance because it is
a vehicle which determines the perception which others have of the

patient, which, in turn, determines how they interact and relate to the patient. The nature of the interaction influences the patient's experience of her illness even if she is elderly, with advanced brain disease. The previous example illustrated the influence of a psychodynamic historical perspective on significant others; the following case demonstrates its influence on the patient.

Mrs. C., an 80-year-old childless widow, sought help because of the recurrence of depression. She possessed a fair amount of insight about factors that influenced her disorder, recognizing a relationship between dark moods and dreams of being scapegoated by her father for family difficulties.

Since early childhood she had distinguished herself in many areas - in ice-skating, her attractive appearance, and excellent job performance. But her father never seemed to recognize her achievements, instead, finding minor faults to criticize. Nonetheless, the patient was proud of her interesting experiences and accomplishments. She took much satisfaction in describing them to me and in registering my positive reactions.

As a young woman, while living in Hollywood, she found herself competing for beaux with some of the early starlets of the silver screen. Mary Pickford was a competitor for one of the men, and Mrs. C. lost that competition. Eventually, she married and settled into a steady, white-collar job.

By age 65, she was a widow and developed an urge for a basic change in life. Always having been an outstanding driver at the wheel of an automobile, she took a job which she described as "a chauffeur for rich ladies". Here, as in all her activities, she demonstrated considerable energy and devotion. To protect these "fine women," she explained, she clandestinely "packed a pistol". Mrs. C. continued this work for about 5 years before, again, going into retirement.

Then, at age 75, experiencing some financial strain, Mrs. C. once more reassessed her diverse skills and resourcefulness and turned to the game of poker with considerable success, in another circle of "rich ladies". By age 80 she had resumed retired life, spending increased time with a new boyfriend. Shortly thereafter, however, she lost the intimacy and companionship of this very dear friend when he died. Feeling suddenly alone, she gradually began to review, and excessively dwell on, her disappointments in life, giving less and less thought to her many satisfying experiences. The ensuing depression eventually led her to seek the aid of a psychiatrist.

She responded well to therapy and took a big leap back into health
several months later, when she struck up a close relationship with
another man. She giggled over her awareness of a general pattern that
she seemed to follow in choosing close male companions; for the most
part they were older men, and she wondered whether this reflected a
longstanding wish to somehow resolve the ambivalent feelings she still
had for her father. This most recent romance was no exception, as she
had begun dating a 97-year-old man. With the continued remission of
her depression, we terminated therapy.

Three years later, I received most distressing news Mrs. C. had
suffered a major stroke, leaving her severely demented. She was
placed in a nursing home, where I went to visit her. Upon arriving
there, I was stunned by what I saw. Instead of being the center of
attraction as she always had, Mrs. C. looked as if she was now the
source of aggravation. Intellectual dysfunction, agitation, and a
high level of disability had made her quite difficult to manage. I
was struck by the matter-of-factness with which the staff walked by
her, with minimal visual contact. This was in such contrast to the
attention she had commanded throughout life. The double tragedy
experienced by the patient in relation to her history, her identity,
became apparent. The first tragedy was more obvious - the break with,
and distance from, her own history, and her inability to access her
own past, due to marked memory impairment. The second, less obvious
tragedy, was the distance she experienced from others, resulting from
their inability to know about the interesting history and vibrant
inner life which she could no longer convey.

We all have a compound history, a two-faceted history - a history as
we ourselves know it and a history as others know it. Not to be
really known by others, to be, in effect, without history because of
an inability to relate one's past, puts us at a severe disadvantage in
eliciting the understanding and empathy of others. Part of the
essence of the human condition is lost. This is the plight of many
patients with advanced dementia. In such situations, the clinician
can be enormously helpful by conveying to the caregivers the
individual's personal and dynamic history, his or her clinical
biography.

In Mrs. C.'s case, an attempt was made to restore some of the
magnetism that accompanies this most human of human phenomena - the
personal history, the biography. Scrapbooks, photos, news clippings
and other important memorabilia were gathered, in an attempt to
dynamically reconstruct a sense of Mrs. C.'s past for the staff. The
impact was pronounced. Upon returning the next week, I observed
noticeably more verbal and non-verbal engagement of the staff with the

patient. As more time passed, it became apparent that, in addition to the staff feeling more in touch with the patient, because they were more in touch with her personal history, they were able to better understand fragments of Mrs. C.'s disjointed thoughts, due to the enlarged frame of reference in which they were heard. Though the magnitude of her dementia was unaltered, Mrs. C.'s agitation diminished. As her connection with others improved so did the quality of her life.

The problem of imparting her history was somewhat complicated because of 2 difficulties - there was more than one shift of personnel each day and there was substantial staff turnover (a particular problem with nursing assistants at nursing homes) during the course of the year.

In a practical manner, how can one effectively convey a patient's history in the dynamic manner described with Mrs. C., for each shift and for new staff? Certainly, it is difficult to achieve this effect via a typical chart history; the length involved might discourage many from reading it. For some institutions, resources are available to develop a program of audiovisual histories. In other settings, if costs are prohibitive, audio-cassette histories could still be feasible. The staff on all shifts might then be much more likely to obtain these histories, due to ease of access - listening to or watching a cassette presentation, as opposed to pondering over a chart. Such a process could also facilitate case conferences or dialogue about the patient among staff viewing or listening to the tapes together.

Family members can also assume an important role in conveying the patient's life story to the staff and derive much satisfaction by contributing to the information and presentation on the cassettes. Particularly if a given family member is a good story-teller, that person should be involved in giving the patient's biography. The experience can be rewarding for all.

To an extent, this last case example demonstrates that, in patients with severe dementia, the role of biography can be as important as that of biology in the overall approach to treatment. It also shows that the opportunity for psychodynamic approaches need not be dismissed by the patient being elderly, by the patient being in a nursing home, or by the patient being brain diseased.

REFERENCES

Altschuler, K.Z., Barad, M. and Goldfarb, A.I. (1963). A survey of dreams in the aged, II, Non-institutionalized subjects. Arch. Gen. Psychiatry, 8, 33-37.

Bondareff, W., Mountjoy, C.Q., Roth, M., Rossor, M.N., Iversen, L.L., Reynolds, G.P. and Hauser, D.L. (1987). Neuronal degeneration in locus ceruleus and cortical correlates of Alzheimer's disease. Alz. Dis. Assoc. Dis., 1(4), 256-262.

Brink, T.L. (1979). Geriatric Psychotherapy. New York: Human Sciences Press.

Brody, E.M. (1986). Informal support systems in the rehabilitation of the disabled elderly. In Brody, J.S., and Ruff, G.E. (eds.). Aging and Rehabilitation. New York: Springer Publishing Company, 87-103.

Cohen, G.D. (1984). The mental health professional and the Alzheimer patient. Hospital and Community Psychiatry, 35, 115-116.

Cohen, G.D. (1985). Psychotherapy with an eighty-year old patient. In Nemiroff, R.A. and Colarusso, C.A. (eds.). The Race Against Time. New York: Plenum Press.

Gallagher, D. (1987). Caregivers of chronically ill elders. In Maddox, G.L. (ed.). Encyclopedia of Aging. New York: Springer.

Gelfand, R. (1980). Glossary. In Kaplan, H.I., Freedman, A.M. and Sadock, B.J. (eds.). Comprehensive Textbook of Psychiatry/III. Baltimore: Williams & Wilkins.

Goldfarb, A.I. and Turner, H. (1953). Psychotherapy of aged persons: utilization and effectiveness of brief therapy. Am. J. Psychiatry, 109, 916-921.

Goldfarb, A.I. and Sheps, J. (1954). Psychotherapy of the aged. Psychosom. Med., 16, 209-219.

Goldstein, K. (1942). Aftereffects of Brain Injuries In War and Their Evaluation and Treatment. New York: Grune and Stratton.

Grotjahn, J.M. (1940). Psychoanalytic investigation of a 71 year old man with senile dementia. Psychoana. Quart., 9, 80-97.

Group for the Advancement of Psychiatry (1988). The Psychiatric Treatment of Alzheimer's Disease. New York: Brunner/Mazel.

Hollos, S. and Ferenczi, S. (1925). Psychoanalysis And The Psychic Disorder Of General Paresis. New York: Nervous and Mental Disease.

Mace, N.L. and Rabins, P.V. (1981). The 36-Hour Day. Baltimore: The Johns Hopkins University Press.

Merriam, A.E., Aronson, M.K., Gaston, P., Wey, S., and Katz, I. (1988). The psychiatric symptoms of Alzheimer's disease. J. Am. Geriatr. Soc., 36, 7-12.

Nathan, R.J., Rose-Itkoff, C. and Lord, G. (1981). Dreams, first memories, and brain atrophy in the elderly. Hillside J. Clin. Psychiatry, 3(2), 139-148.

Reifler, B.V. and Larson, E. (1988). Excess disability in demented elderly outpatients: The rule of halves. J. Am. Geriatr. Soc., 36, 82-83.

Reifler, B.V, Larson, E., Teri, L. and Poulsen, M. (1986). Dementia of the Alzheimer's type and depression. J. Am. Geriatr. Soc., 34, 855-859.

Steury, S. and Blank, M.L. (eds.), (1977). Readings in Psychotherapy With Older People. Rockville, Maryland: National Institute of Mental Health.

Teri, L., Larson, E.B. and Reifler, B.V. (1988). Behavioural disturbance in dementia of the Alzheimer's type. J. Am. Geriatr. Soc., 36, 1-6.

U.S. Department of Health and Human Services (1987). Differential diagnosis of dementing diseases. National Institutes of Health Consensus Development Conference Statement, 6(11), 1-27.

Verwoerdt, A. (1981). Individual psychotherapy in senile dementia. In Miller, N.E. and Cohen, G.D. (eds). Clinical Aspects of Alzheimer's Disease and Senile Dementia. New York: Raven Press.

CHAPTER 5

PSYCHOTHERAPY AND THE COGNITIVELY IMPAIRED ELDERLY

Joel Sadavoy, M.D., F.R.C.P.(C)
Anne Robinson, R.N.
Baycrest Centre for Geriatric Care
University of Toronto
Toronto, Ontario

INTRODUCTION

Cognitive decline is often a devastating event, whatever the cause. It assaults the very core of the individual - his or her capacity for reflection and memory, emotional intimacy, love and warmth, giving and receiving advice and respect, and tolerating or taking pleasure in the daily passage of life. Those who care for the slowly disappearing self of their mother, father, sister, or brother, are left puzzled, helpless and, most importantly, progressively less able to communicate. Relationships that have a past of vital interaction gradually evolve into the isolated and painful solitudes of two people deeply connected by history but irrevocably separated by this disease.

One is at times deeply moved by images of a devoted husband, wife, child or sibling, sitting quietly and watchfully beside their loved one who, silent and unreachable, sits behind the veil of their illness. Sometimes, in desperation one of them will attempt to reach out, to make contact, their efforts uncomprehended by the other. Both suffer but neither seem able to comfort - a funeral without an end.

Coupled with the pain and unresolved grief of the lingering, the frustration of the caretaking and the anger caused by the rejection inherent in the illness, are the practical matters of everyday life. How can the impaired and the intact live together? Because those who are ill are so cut off by their disease, caregivers often abandon verbal and emotional interaction. In their place caregivers address the apparently more compelling physical and safety needs of the new patient. This may happen because the overwhelming task for a caregiver is to maintain order in the lives of all who are living together. Frequently, under these circumstances, whatever "self" that remains of the impaired individual

101

fades, his or her illness and its overt effects becoming the overwhelming source of his or her identity. No longer is it easily possible to discern the landmarks of the patient's personality - strength, fears, humour, love; all are submerged beneath the compelling "symptoms" - agitation, forgetfulness, withdrawal, suspicion, repetition.

Love does not always succumb easily to the rejecting illness. A spouse, child or sibling may fight at each juncture to preserve whatever they can of the relationship, sometimes with understanding, and other times with anger and desperation - "try to get dressed and come for a walk; why don't you remember where you put things; I'll never put you in a home." Unfortunately, the well-meaning or desperate efforts to restore what used to be, may not be understood by the patient who reacts with withdrawal, anxiety, or bizarreness. More and more the person fades, seeming out of reach of normal communication.

In the chain of events attached to cognitive decline, strangers become a necessary caregiving resource at some point, at least in the western world. Not only do these new caregivers have to cope with multiple practical problems of daily care for the increasingly dependent, and sometimes demanding patient, they must do so with little or no actual experience of the "person" who lived before the illness. They do not know who it is they care for, at least not at the beginning. With effort some of the patient's story can be learned, but a true empathic experience of the other person, so crucial to depth of caring and such a central need of human life is almost impossible to achieve from the mere written record of a life. What then is the well-motivated caregiver, professional or family to do? In part the answer lies in methods of therapy which emphasize establishing contact with, and reaching out to, the person within the illness. In this way caregivers can learn about the deeper identity of their charges, and extend their efforts beyond simply responding to their overt needs and the demands of daily life.

In this chapter we will briefly review some of the more frequently used therapeutic approaches to the demented elderly but restrict ourselves to those interventions which utilize interactive methods and communication (in its broadest sense). The biological component of treatment of these patients is crucial and must be critically evaluated, however, others have capably addressed that issue elsewhere in this volume. Following a selective review of other work, we will address one central question - what remains of the personality and the self as the mind fragments. To explore this question we will use one case study of an intensive therapeutic relationship. Such detailed clinical descriptions are sparse in the psychotherapy literature of dementia despite the importance of attempting to know and describe the inner experience of the dementing individual. If we can obtain this understanding, we can target our interventions appropriately and avoid using assumption and idiosyncratic, personal opinions to construct management plans.

Each of the approaches to be reviewed here shares one common characteristic - the attempt of a caregiver to influence a patient by verbal or nonverbal interactions, without the primary use of physical or biological interventions. Broadly speaking these approaches may be termed psychotherapies.

We are aware that the divisions of treatment approaches are arbitrary, and often overlapping. This is probably a function of the universality of some human experiences which are difficult or impossible to separate into defined categories. While many approaches strive for purity of technique, the successful ones have one common, non-specific element - the human interaction of a caregiver with a patient.

BEHAVIOURAL AND LEARNING THERAPIES

Behavioural and learning approaches have been extensively applied to the cognitively impaired elderly especially in institutions. As a technique for this group, they focus on specific target behaviours. In most situations these behaviours are identified by the staff. Unlike many other situations in psychiatry, these patients cannot and generally do not have insight into their own problems, nor do they often request change or help with their behaviour. Hence, in the main it is up to others to target "troublesome" problems and institute methods of change, a diagnostic and treatment task requiring great care, understanding and empathy, since it is undertaken unilaterally, without the patient's explicit consent or even cooperation.

In their narrowest applications behaviour therapies may be applied to a single troublesome symptom such as urinary incontinence (Pollock and Liberman, 1974). In their broadest applications, the whole patient, not the symptom, is the focus of therapy. Rather than targeting specific symptoms, treatment has the broader aim of helping patients develop and express their unique interests and strengths. Hussian (1984) has defined the goals of behavioural modification therapy. These include increasing the patient's level of participation in activities, such as recreation, exercise, and other ADL; enhancing the patient's social interest and interactions; improving communication skills and verbal behaviour; and improving performance on concrete tasks - toileting, bathing, ambulation, feeding and noncompliance with routines.

Katz (1976) has pointed out that the factors in the patient which overlie the basic illness (dementia) are amenable to change. While brain

damage is permanent, overall function can be improved. This broad view of
the patient leads Katz to use behavioural therapy as only one element in a
treatment that also utilizes educational, milieu, and activity approaches.
While many factors confound pure research in this area, Katz's study showed
that 44% of 80 treated patients improved, 20% were unchanged, 18% worse and
18% were not rated.

In general, the literature suggests that the gains from pure behaviour
modification approaches in the institutionalized elderly, unassociated with
milieu and other therapies, are not encouraging. Leng's (1982) review
points out the paucity of reports of successful interventions although some
researchers such as Wisner and Green (1986) describe better outcomes.

One problem with behavioural approaches for this group lies in the
external process of goal-setting ie., most frequently the caregivers
decide what is desireable and set up programs to mold behaviour in these
directions. Unfortunately, we still know little about the impact of our
programs on the individual, in part because his/her inner world is so
inaccessible. For example, increased activity levels may seem
advantageous to the patient. But in an individual case is it better, or
does it perhaps raise the patient's inner sense of dysphoria and anxiety?
Therapists must guard against imposing externally created goals based on
subjective views of what "a person" should be. As Harris et al (1977)
point out, these patients are often captive and helpless. They raise the
question of whether and how to gain the patient's consent when setting out
goals and treatment plans.

Reality orientation, based on a learning model, has been used
extensively, especially in institutions. The main goal of this therapy is
to preserve or improve the patient's orientation through various
educational and reinforcing techniques. These fall broadly into two
categories - a classroom type approach wherein a group leader presents to
and elicits from the patients, relevant personal and environmental
orienting information. The second approach requires staff to adopt a
reality reinforcing approach twenty-four hours a day whenever they have
patient contact. Frequently such programs are highly structured,
requiring carefully designed staff responses to patient behaviours.

Results are mixed. Overall, the more interactive and "person
centered" the interventions, the greater the improvement. Hanley, McGuire
and Boyd (1981) showed no effect from classroom approaches, but dramatic
improvement from the 24 hour approach. Harris and Ivory (1976) commented
on the promising results from reality orientation therapy, although noting
that behaviour per se is little changed. More striking was the improvement
in orientation and reduction in bizarre speech. Holden and Sinebruchow
(1978) suggested that reality orientation is a technique that attracts the

attention and enthusiasm of the staff, and, as such, helps to structure the staff's responses, thereby making them more comfortable with their patients. Harris et al (1977) described more generalized effects from reality orientation with improved verbal behaviour, social interaction, and physical activity and reduced self-injurious behaviour. However, in Leng's (1982) review of behavioural treatment of the elderly he concluded that the overall gains from reality orientation are, unfortunately, modest at best and generally not sustained.

One of the crucial questions of technique is the relationship between the application of behavioural theory and the realities of staff-patient and staff-staff interaction. As already noted, behavioural therapies often rely on specific theories and heavily structured techniques which pay little heed to the interaction of residents and staff that are "extraneous" to the treatment plan. In an excellent study of a unit utilizing behavioural therpy, Buckholdt and Gubrium (1983) examined other factors in ward life impacting on the treatment but not considered part of the behavioural treatment plan. They called these factors "the underlife" of the caregivers on an institutional unit. Underlife refers to the tacit understandings, common sense reasoning, negotiations among professionals, ad hoc procedures and intuitive decision-making amongst staff which are not explicitly defined as a component of the behavioural management program for the unit. Buckholdt and Gubrium suggest that staff trained in reality orientation often remain fixed on behaviour, rely strictly on reality orientation interventions and avoid talking with the patient or listening to their words. Although these staff-patient and staff-staff interactions occur on every unit, these authors suggest that such "underlife" factors are ignored and not considered since they are outside the behavioural model. They go on to question the theoretical adequacy of a behavioural model that fails to address the underlife factors of social organization and interaction surrounding therapeutic application.

Despite the many cautions implied by the literature on behavioural therapies, these approaches offer important therapeutic modalities which, when combined with an awareness of staff, milieu and interpersonal factors, can be of central practical value. Indeed, the behaviour of demented patients is sometimes inaccessible to any other therapeutic interventions. However, in geriatric therapy pure "formulistic" approaches of any kind, whether organic, psychological or social are generally confounded by the complexity of the illnesses that are being treated. This helps to explain why the role of group process and the development of close consistent staff-patient involvement arises repeatedly in descriptions of behavioural interventions, (Brook, Degund and Mather, 1975) and why it has been pointed out that, while many techniques may alter behaviour, the content of the program may be less important then the structured contact of staff with patients (Citrin and Dixon, 1977).

GROUP THERAPY

Group therapies have been the preferred mode of therapeutic intervention for the cognitively impaired. Whether these groups are formal therapy - psychotherapy, psychodrama, exercise, activity, current events and so on, or non-specific groups - the ward or unit as a whole - demented patients are rarely dealt with individually. The basic wisdom of this therapeutic attitude is not readily apparent, nor has there been any convincing work to establish the usefulness of group approaches as opposed to individual interventions. Clearly, groups seem more efficient and have the inherent advantage of bringing relatively isolated individuals into contact with others. However, one may also suspect that the group setting distances the therapist/caregiver from the individual patient, and thereby relieves some of the burden, anxiety and perhaps boredom of having to confront the often difficult personalities of the cognitively impaired on a one to one basis.

The more common types of groups focus on exercise, socialization and daily living tasks, (Allen, 1976; Aronson, Levin and Lipkowitz, 1984; Berger, 1978; Katz, 1976) less frequently dealing with inner feeling, this, despite reports of some very positive results using psychodynamic groups with impaired elderly institutionalized patients (Akerlund and Norberg, 1986; Cox, 1985; Lazarus, 1976; Linden, 1953; Silver, 1950). Linden (1953) for example, concluded that, in a setting of acceptance, interested care, and creative participation, old values regain their importance, hunger for social relationships returns, regression is halted and an urge to contribute to group cohesion emerges.

Akerlund and Norberg (1986) reported an array of therapeutic responses in demented patients seen in psychodynamically oriented group therapy, including the presence of traditional resistance and psychological defences, transference and countertransference manifestations. Cox (1985) used group therapy to help cognitively impaired patients deal with intimate feelings in a consciously constructed environment of open communication and confidentiality. The aim, in contrast to behavioural approaches, was to change attitudes toward self and others rather than behaviour. The goal was to help the patient experience a more tangible meaning to life, by promoting trust, acceptance and a sense of belonging.

Most reports of verbal and interactional group approaches confirm their humanizing impact on institutionalized, demented patients. For example, Manaster (1972), using a social format, described the development of a group's capacity to safely criticize and to become more challenging, spontaneous and focused. Yalom and Terrazas (1968) noted that, particularly with uninvolved or withdrawn (although not specifically cognitively impaired) patients evidence of increased closeness or intimacy develops late in the life of a group. Lazarus (1976) commented on problems in implementing group psychotherapy with this patient population including the threat of a group to previously withdrawn patients, patients' jealousy of each other and a wish for special attention from the leaders. Overall, group therapists with this population must be patient and content to measure change in relatively small increments.

As with much of the psychotherapy literature these studies are largely uncontrolled and anecdotal. Moreover, while the work takes place in long-term care institutions and with patients of varying degrees of cognitive intactness, precise definition of the patient population including the type of dementia and its severity are lacking. Despite these limitations, however, this work remains instructive for those who treat demented elderly.

MILIEU THERAPY

Undoubtedly, the commonest "psychotherapeutic" approach to the cognitively impaired elderly is "milieu therapy". Some programs are informal, while others are more thoughtful and structured. However, virtually any custodial unit, chronic hospital or home for the aged makes some efforts in this direction. Almost all reports of these approaches are positive about outcome and conclude that there has been generalized improvement (Allen, 1976; Charatan, 1980; Berger, 1978; Gottesman, Quarterman and Cohn, 1973; Hussian, 1984; Manaster, 1972; McEvoy and Patterson, 1986; Miller, 1977; Cameron, 1941; Cosin et al, 1958; Brody et al, 1974; Reichenfeld et al, 1973; Roskos, Lerner and Kline, 1979; Schafer, 1985; Schwab, Rader and Doan, 1985; Whyte, Constantopoulos and Bevans, 1982).

Techniques of milieu therapy vary widely but generally incorporate elements of normalizing life through social activity, exercise, music, physical contact, activities of daily living, gardening, and so on. Often, reality orientation and behavioural approaches are incorporated. Most programs are implemented by nursing staff. The precise roles of the other members of the much-vaunted multidisciplinary team are described vaguely.

The goals of milieu approaches are diverse and include improved self-esteem, relaxation, exercise, social involvement and participation, improved communication skills, and improved activities of daily living.

Brody et al (1971) attempted a more specific study of which aspects of their patients' behaviour could be expected to change under the impact of an intensive, individualized, milieu treatment program. The concept of excess disability introduced by Kahn (1965) is central here. Excess disability refers to the discrepency which exists between the individual's actual functional incapacity and the incapacity one would expect to be produced by the impairment.

This study population was severely mentally and physically impaired, institutionalized aged, living in a sophisticated custodial setting. The treatment was individualized and multidisciplinary and it focused on the multiplicity of disabilities of the patient and the setting of realistic goals for change. Observations were objective and utilized a battery of rating scales. Seven categories of excess disabilities were identified for each patient and targeted for specific therapy. Final patient evaluations were made after one year.

The seven categories of excess disability which were evaluated were mobility, self care, social relationships, family relationships, organized activity, individualized activity, and emotional discomfort. Only two items of the seven categories seemed influenced by the treatment program; family relationships and individualized activities showed statistically significant improvement. Overall, the investigators judged the experimental group to be improved, in comparison to controls and confirmed that certain excess disabilities can be ameliorated with treatment. Equally important, the study confirmed the need to identify those factors which can be altered by therapy and separate them from the vast majority of patient factors which remain unaffected by comprehensive therapy.

FAMILY THERAPY

One of the mainstays of therapy for the cognitively impaired is supportive and educational therapy for their families and caregivers. A detailed discussion of this modality is beyond the scope of this chapter since it is therapy targeted at the family rather than the patient, but, the value of this work is undisputable (Aronson, Levin and Lipkowitz, 1984; Barnes et al, 1981; Brane, 1986; Eisdorfer and Cohen, 1981; Gwyther and Blazer, 1984; Haley, 1983; LaVorgna, 1979; Lazarus et al, 1981; Levine, Dastoor and Gendron, 1983; Levine et al, 1984; Mann, 1986; Ratna and Davis, 1984; Schmidt and Keyes, 1985; Teusink and Mahler, 1984). It is interesting to note that the patient is rarely involved, either as a member of family group therapy or as a participant in any level of planning. Of course we all recognize the frequent inability of the patient to be a full participant, but the evidence from group therapy in institutions indicates their capacity to "feel" involved and express feelings. Once again, the caution must be voiced for therapists to beware of avoiding contact with the patient and rationalizing that their illness will prevent them from meaningful participation.

INDIVIDUAL PSYCHOTHERAPY

Individual psychotherapy for the cognitively impaired elderly is a rare phenomenon, if one is to judge from reports in the literature. Few detailed case reports of such therapy are recorded although some articles hint that this type of work may occur, although it goes largely unreported.

Goldfarb (Goldfarb and Turner, 1953; Goldfarb and Sheps, 1954; Goldfarb, 1967) was an early pioneer in the use of individual psychotherapy for the institutionalized elderly. His approach focused on the need of such patients for a sense of control over forces beyond their power to change. The technique of therapy encouraged an idealizing transference, thereby permitting the patient to "borrow" the therapist's power and prestige, and reducing his/her feeling of helplessness. Additionally, the patient's sense of power was further reinforced by allowing him/her to "win" in certain arenas of control, fostering an illusion of overcoming the powerful therapist. Goldfarb reported that this method was effective in reducing behavioural and anxiety symptoms. It took only 15 minutes, one session, weekly. Despite the usefulness of this approach (which used principles that anticipated self-psychology and its application to the aged (Lazarus, 1980)) detailed descriptions and in-depth understanding of the inner world of the patient remained absent from the reports.

A second "specific" technique of geriatric psychotherapy, life-review, was first developed by Butler (1963). While not specifically intended for the cognitively impaired elderly, life-review and its relative, reminiscence, have been promoted for use with this patient group (Allen, 1976; Charatan, 1980). Often, a group setting is the forum used and reminiscing or life-review groups abound. Similarly, its use is frequent in individual therapy and often effective, although on a cautionary note, it may also be a convenient method for an uncertain therapist to avoid true engagement with the patient. Additionally, Lawton (1975), supported by Merriam (1980) and Ackerlund and Norberg (1986), suggested that life-review is often stressful, and that no particular support or therapeutic advantage is seen for a strategy of directing the older person toward life-review behaviour. A similar caution was raised in a previous paper in reference to characterologically disturbed patients (Sadavoy, 1987). Lesser et al (1981) found that reminiscing was primarily an early phenomenon of group psychotherapy. While it apparently served as a bridge between early group uncertainty and later stages of trust, intimacy and openness, it tended to diminish when the group became more cohesive. Despite these cautions, reminiscence is an evident human need which, if used appropriately, avoiding formulistic applications, helps to create contact and warmth with others, as well as reinforcing inner self-cohesion.

Lazarus, Cohler and Lesser are among the first to examine the nature of personality change in Alzheimer's disease. Specifically they ask what happens to personal integrity, the individual's sense of continuity over space and time, morale and well-being. They note the increased (and perhaps normative) orientation to inner experience (interiority) during the early period of old age, while reliance on life-review as a predominant mode of psychological coping emerges only in the eighth or ninth decade.

Life review, the authors conclude, represents the patient's attempt and need to maintain psychological order and continuity of the self. By incorporating both object relations and self psychology theory, this process can be seen as a normal psychological method to preserve self-integration by maintaining the intrapsychologic experience of others - the "evoked other" in Stern's terms. In other words, through recall and reminiscence of significant others, a sense of self-cohesion and solace is preserved.

Unfortunately Alzheimer's patients generally have specific problems with verbal and abstract expression. Their normal reminiscing "defense" may be impaired, and confused, and difficult for both the patient and observer to comprehend. How then can one tap into their inner experience? Lazarus et al suggest the use of the empathic method to get inside ie., use of intuition and empathic rapport by experienced therapists thereby tuning into the patients' essential experience.

They thus undertook a 5 year study of 53 Alzheimer's patients to rate the fragmentation of the self using a self-psychology rating scale administered by a group of experienced clinicians. Not surprisingly, compared to the 47 healthy controls, the SDAT (senile dementia Alzheimer's type) sufferers showed a greater difficulty in maintaining personality integration. The results of the study suggest that these demented patients are more sensitive to empathic failures, than non-demented subjects, a finding supported by the case study to follow.

The implications are important. If one accepts this evidence, therapists will have to recognize that these patients require greater individual efforts to "know" them and their specific self-sustaining needs. Individual personal relationships then become crucial to the preservation of their maximum self-integration. Therapists must guard against acceptance of withdrawal and incapacity as inevitable (Steuer, 1982; Linden, 1957), and avoid the common practice of treating these patients only in groups, and avoiding individual contact.

CASE STUDY

Therapists are oriented to change and cure and that is as it should be. But before therapy must come understanding. The case which follows is presented in that spirit. Whether the understanding gleaned, the techniques used or the results obtained should or can be generalized must be left an open question. The goal of this case examination is only to help explore the inner world of a progressively dementing woman as it was revealed in her unique relationship to a therapist, who sat and talked with her, once a week, for 4 years.

Sara A's History

The patient, Sara A., was born in 1899 near Kiev in Russia, the younger of 2 girls. Her early life is known to her therapist only through her own memories, which were invariably poignant. Her mother died when she was 8 years old. She has only one reported memory of her mother, who was lying in bed ill. Crying, she said to her young daughter "I don't want to die, help me!" Sara's memories of her father are of a tall, handsome "lady's man". She remembers him as a loving father, who personally taught her to read and encouraged her. However, 6 months after her mother's death, her father remarried. The patient's stepmother was, in the patient's memory, a caricature of the wicked stepmother - physically abusive, favoring her own 6 children (Sara's half siblings), demanding of Sara and her sister. She hated her stepmother who remained a vibrant inner psychic figure for the patient, into old age. Even in the grip of the dementing process, as we will see, wicked uncaring mothers were a constant preoccupation, and focus of her delusions.

The patient remembered her longing for her father each time he left on financially necessary but prolonged trips. One recurring powerful snapshot is of Sara, a little girl, standing peering out the window into the darkness, desperate for her father's return, in terror that he would not come, abandoning her to her hated stepmother.

Sara's one potential childhood ally, her sister, was a disappointment. Perhaps in response to the unavoidable neglect and absence of love, rivalry rather than support characterized their relationship. In Sara's memory her sister felt responsible for her, but resentful. Indeed, when it came time to leave Europe, Sara, aged 15, left first to join her grandmother in Canada using a ticket meant for her sister. Her sister's jealousy was further fueled by her younger sister marrying before she, the eldest. The strain and distance in that relationship never healed, even after Sara saved for and sent passage to Canada for her sister and subsequently arranged a job for her. In her mind, her sister remained angry and disappointed in her to the end.

After emigration at the age of 17, Sara married and had 2 daughters of her own. Her personality makeup was never fully revealed to the therapist, but it is clear that she was a highly anxious, albeit self-sacrificing, mother. Her focus, not surprisingly in light of her own losses, was on the safety of her children. She worried constantly that something would happen to them. In the midst of economic hardship (they earned little, she as a seamstress, he a carpenter) the patient maintained a stable orthodox religious home. In her public life the patient was a friendly, well-liked woman active in community affairs and president of a local volunteer chapter.

Both daughters married young. The elder twice divorced, the younger happily married. The elder daughter had been in lifelong conflict with her mother and echoed Sara's fearful insecurity. Her children (Sara's grandchildren) had shown instability and Sara was preoccupied with their safety and happiness. When she was 62, Sara's husband died. After several years of taking in boarders to support herself, she remarried to a quiet man with whom she spent a few happy years, with travel, friendships and shared pleasures. Unfortunately, when 76 years old, Sara developed Parkinson's disease. Three years later, following a series of falls, she began to decline precipitously and she was admitted to an old age home for care.

Following admission Sara had a difficult and stormy course. Initially she reacted with "depression" and a sense of being trapped and abandoned. As time passed her depression deepened and she developed delusions. It was this course which lead to a request for help from the psychiatric consultation team. The initial assessment revealed that Sara had extensive delusions that her grandchildren were dead and that she too should die. Successful pharmacological therapy (amitriptyline 35 mg q.h.s. and thioridazine 10 mg q.h.s.) settled the worst of her agitation and weekly psychotherapy began. Throughout the next 4 years, the nurse clinician (A.R.), an experienced psycho-therapist, supervised weekly by a psychiatrist spoke to Sara in weekly formal sessions approximately 30-45 minutes long. Although the patient's condition fluctuated, it was punctuated by exacerbations in her delusions and agitation, and showed a gradual progressive cognitive decline with deepening memory loss, disorientation and confusion, aphasia, apraxia, and emotional lability.

The therapeutic vignettes to follow will help to chart the development of this unique therapeutic relationship and its stormy, but revealing, course.

The therapist's first task was to decide whether this patient was an appropriate person to see regularly. She needed several assessment interviews to verify first, Sara's capacity to generate a rapport in the interviews and second that she was soothed and comforted by the contact and discussions. The capacity to be soothed by the presence of a *specific* other is a central indication for ongoing regular contact between patient and therapist. Finally, Sara showed an ability to utilize verbal interaction, unlike more debilitated and impaired individuals who often require more basic communication, for example in the form of touch and motion.

From the outset, both therapist and supervisor recognized that some special therapeutic skills were required in this case. The therapist had to be able to tolerate the patient's free form, often unfocused thoughts, while continuing to maintain an inquiring stance in relationship to the material - that is, an ongoing attempt to translate the words into a form that further enhanced the under-standing of the patient's inner world. She had to recognize that the patient's logic would often be different from hers. While this is true in all psychotherapy, it is especially so when the patient is capable of only minimal corrective feedback to the therapist, i.e. to correct the therapist's inevitable mistakes of understanding. Moreover, because of Sara's severely limited memory, the therapist had the task of maintaining continuity between sessions. Finally, when Sara's delusions began to incorporate the therapist, she had to have the ability to tolerate this often difficult experience without undue anxiety, overcorrection or withdrawal. Examples of these difficulties abound. Sara, for instance, early in the relationship, began to refuse food. She was convinced the food had been made from the severed limbs of her children and the children of her therapist. She accused the therapist of making this hideous stew. The therapist, rather than correcting the "facts" recognized the patient's inner terror and feelings of vulnerability. She remembered Sara's early history of violence and loss and she simply said that those thoughts must be very frightening. She did not share the content of the delusions with the other staff at that time, since this would only have fuelled their labelling of Sara as crazy.

Throughout the early months of contact, Sara's themes were consistent. She feared her grandchildren were being left uncared for (a projection of her early experience) and that they would be killed (perhaps reflecting her childhood fears of her stepmother's violence). The therapist responded that, while those things had not happened, Sara must be very frightened, as though after a bad dream. Interestingly as time passed Sara began to preface her comments with "I had one of those dreams" and on one occasion "I screamed for you but you weren't there".

Sara's desperate inner turmoil was accentuated by her growing cognitive impairment. She could not report the day, time, or her location. She seemed to have no memory of visitors and was often severely agitated. She would bang and rattle her bed, scream and shout demeaning epithets at staff. She was paranoid and accused her roommate of "peeing" on her clothes - "then they smell and nobody likes me". Sara herself was incontinent and had an awareness, albeit distorted, of her odor and perhaps shame.

Despite Sara's frequent states of apparent chaos, the therapist's presence routinely settled and calmed her. This was so until the day the therapist took notes overtly for the first time. "You're putting things in the paper about me" accused Sara. "They were things I only told you and so I know it's you". It was then that a prolonged angry rejecting phase of therapy began (perhaps we can call this a negative transference, albeit psychotic). Sara accused the therapist of being a bad mother to her children. She said she knew this because her daughter had told her in a "dream" that the therapist's children were suffering.

While we must be cautious not to overinterpret this material with too much conviction, it is possible that we were witnessing the raw and primitive response of Sara to a momentary lapse of empathy by the therapist. Unable to control or modulate her disappointment, nor deal with it with the therapist in reality, her unresolved rage and grief at her mother abandoning her took over and was projected into the relationship. In the resultant projective identification Sara took on the familiar role and emotions of the mistreated lonely child and the therapist became her mother or perhaps the hated feared stepmother.

Another interesting theme was Sara's concern that she would be evicted from the home. This feeling arose during a period when the staff had attempted to confront Sara's delusions, telling her, for example, that nobody was stealing from her. Sara became predictably more agitated and yelled at the nurses. Later she told her therapist - "the nurses won't come in now because I'm bad, I say crazy things". Then she asked for reassurance that her grandchildren were not dead, killed because of the bad things she'd done.

What is most fascinating is that this insight and discussion came from a woman who, at the time, was unable to recognize her own written name. Clearly, whatever the degree of dementia, levels of interpersonal awareness remained, albeit intermittently.

Other islands of insight were revealed in the transference. Sara clearly saw the therapist as a strong and reliable figure. She said "I can tell you these things, but don't tell my daughter. She gets too upset". The strength and reliability of a therapist is of great importance to a vulnerable patient, an observation made long ago by Goldfarb (Goldfarb and Turner, 1953; Goldfarb, 1967; Goldfarb and Sheps, 1954). It is further bolstered by consistent performance by the therapist - regularity of appointments, maintenance of confidentiality (even though the patient may never know the difference) and loyalty to the patient's welfare. As we observed above, this patient, like others with similar problems, was exquisitely sensitive to change (taking notes) and responded with a paranoid storm that took three weeks to abate. A further instructive element of Sara's relationship to reality was revealed during these delusional episodes. On the one hand Sara clearly reacted with rage and paranoid hurt if the therapist disappointed her, for example, by going away on vacation. On the other hand, Sara maintained a double bookkeeping system (splitting perhaps) wherein she continued to trust the therapist, ask for her help and identify with her "You must be Jewish like me" she said. Almost simultaneously she would say "You are publishing my thoughts and destroying my family" and then "I was waiting for you to come" (the time of that session had been changed that day). In passing it's worth realizing that Sara had recognized and remembered, albeit dimly, that something (the time of the session) had changed. But she was unable to fully understand what had happened. All she could experience was a vague unfocused anxiety leading to increased agitation. The implication for technique here, is that it is as important or perhaps more so, to be scrupulous about issues of time and regularity. With the cognitively impaired, one may erroneously rationalize that the patient won't realize or remember. Clearly this is often not true and can precipitate aberrant behaviour. Unwary staff can easily miss the causal connections and attribute the behaviour to spontaneous "craziness".

As noted earlier, the relationship between a dementing patient and a therapist is maintained by tenuous links. The thread of a relationship may be sustained by a momentary indication of trust that the therapist will not be shocked by the patients' thoughts. In Sara's words - "We've always told each other the truth". The therapist recognized her need to talk about herself. Her thoughts were so bizarre,

however, that no one would take them seriously. Most others saw her
pain as craziness and responded to her as bothersome or assaultive.

The therapist's tolerance of the patient is of special importance. In
Sara's case, she was the only one who could remain with the patient.
Sara's daughters ran in and out on visits, in self preservation and
often the staff did the same. As I have tried to show, Sara remained
aware of how others recoiled from her, especially her family.

In the second year of therapy the relationship was a central force in
Sara's life. The therapist was strongly incorporated into Sara's
inner world. Because of her impairment, the expression of conflict
was raw and unmodified often involving the therapist in a primitive
transference. For example in one session Sara said "If my mother were
here she would have loved you". Then later - "I didn't think you'd
have the nerve to come. I can't believe you helped to kill them.
They say (a hallucination or dream) that girl (the therapist) you love
so much talked about you". Then "I think so much of her (therapist)
that I can say anything to you". We see here how Sara's inner world
of longing, fear, loss and rage are expressed in free floating
projections - her strong positive feelings alternating with paranoid
fear.

The therapist noted these oscillations and as well became aware of how
Sara's confusion would flow over her from one moment to the next. She
would begin to stare intently at the therapist as though to establish
who she was and then suddenly withdraw into an eyes-closed reverie.
Both patient and therapist had to struggle with what was confusion,
delusion, and hallucination, and what was reality.

The bridge to reality is often difficult to maintain. The therapist
facilitated this by encouraging reminiscence to overcome the gaps of
understanding. As the therapist said, "This was the only way I could
fill in the part of the person that was missing from the demented
patient". She also used her own reality and gave personal (but
relevant) information about herself to Sara. At times when Sara
drifted too far from reality and did not return, the therapist brought
her back to the here and now by orienting her. This was not to
admonish or correct her but to reestablish contact at that moment.
When Sara would close her eyes and ramble in her delusions the
therapist broke in with - "Sara, I'm A.R. I'm a nurse and I'm here to
talk to you".

As time passed, Sara's themes remained consistent - killing, abandoned
children, poor mothering. However, it is a crucial observation that
her delusions sprang from the interplay of her memories and early life

experience with her current everyday interactive experience. For example, when the nurses walked away from her as they often did, she responded by screaming "Help me". We can understand this plea most usefully if we see it as an amalgam of her immediate sense of helpless which had resurrected her earlier abandonment experiences. This perspective suggests that the delusions of dementia are not just concrete misinterpretations of reality (eg., my clothes smell someone must have tried to poison me). The evidence from this case shows the strong presence of early life experience in the verbal and emotional productions of the patient.

In year III Sara remembered her mother's death when she was 8 years old. She was recounting again how she came to Canada, her guilt over taking her sister's ticket and then her mother. "I said to my mother (shouting) Don't die! and she died". This massive return of painful memory came with the power and freshness of an immediate moment. Then she told how she became the mother - had to cook and clean and be a mother when she was only eight. It was then that she spoke of waiting at the window at end of day for her father's return.

In year IV despite increasing forgetfulness and in a moment of clarity, Sara wrote this poem:

> My eyes are not good
> I can't read and I can't write
> I have no hope to get better
> I try my best but I can't remember things
> I still hope, I still hope that time will help me,
> I am old
> I cry a lot

By the end of year IV, the therapist no longer saw Sara with regularity. She was too demented, had lost all capacity to connect. Her therapist had seen her virtually every Tuesday for four years. Sara died 1½ years later completely demented and in an essentially vegetative state.

Central to understanding this relationship is recognizing the impact Sara's treatment had on her therapist. The therapist became quickly attached to the frail, tiny, well-mannered Sara and learned to understand and deal with the psychotic, rambling, accusing Sara. As time passed, Sara became frailer, but the therapist and supervisor realized that she was too concerned with her patient's state. The therapist spontaneously began to explore the reasons for her feelings, which she discovered were rooted in powerful countertransference reactions. These stemmed from longstanding ideas she held about her own parents. As she came to know Sara's conflicts she began to see her parent's behaviour in a new perspective, one which caused her to recognize their separateness as individuals. Not only were they her parents they were people with a past who struggled with conflicts often unrelated to her, their child. As she understood these realities, the therapist began to question her lifelong assumptions about her parents and herself. She saw Sara's daughters recapitulating their mother's early experiences in their own lives and began to see the danger of the same type of repetition in her life.

In her words she said "I don't know my parents anymore, I only know the myths I've created about them". Other countertransference reactions developed. The therapist saw herself as Sara's only ally and wanted to become the good daughter (and mother) and to be different from Sara's unavailable daughters. In time she also realized her wish to be loved by Sara. This was a difficult time, because Sara was incapable of such responses. On the contrary, the therapist had to deal with Sara's psychotic often vicious accusations of betrayal and abandonment. These projections drew the therapist into a chaotic emotional world of primary process which frequently left her wondering "Is she crazy or am I?". These feelings are akin to those of therapists who encounter the primitive projections of borderline or psychotic patients in psychotherapy.

In analyzing this case, therapist and supervisor considered the role of the other staff in the therapeutic system. Recognizing the temptation to view staff as the bad objects and "defend" Sara against them, the therapist drew them into the process. She used their observations of Sara's behaviour, spoke to them about her findings and became allied with them in their struggle to deal with and help Sara. However, as noted above, she was selective about certain pieces of information. She tried to help them reformulate Sara's behaviour into understandable terms, as one does with other difficult patients (Book, Sadavoy and Silver, 1978). Sara's behaviour had to be translated from "bad" to troubled. She formulated specific behaviours - eg., her crying out for help as an expression of a child's pain. The therapist helped make Sara a whole person for the staff by sharing her history with them. Together they worked out new and practical measures of intervention based on their newly acquired understanding of the patient. For eg., How to soothe her by sitting with her; helping staff to refrain from imposing their "rational" views on Sara, an approach she often experienced as assaultive. Despite the challenge of Sara's behaviour they lived with her for 6½ years until her death. She was never transferred to the special-care dementia ward, as are so many other difficult dementing patients.

This case demonstrates the richness of experience one can derive by forming an intense relationship with another person whose cognition is gradually receding. Sara showed us how dementia may destroy the defensive barriers to unconscious life and release repressed unmodified memories. The result is an overwhelming flood of chaotic psychotic regression. It was clear that only by minutely understanding the intricate tapestry of memory, feeling, personality and distortion which made up the fabric of the patient's newly formed demented persona, could the therapist tease out the patient's reality and respond with care and humanity.

PRACTICAL APPROACHES TO COMMUNICATING WITH THE COGNITIVELY IMPAIRED PATIENT

Assessment For Psychotherapy

History

As Gene Cohen illustrated in his chapter, a central component of the therapeutic process is a thorough and sensitive knowledge of the patient's identity as an individual, separate and apart from his/her disease. The preceeding clinical example illustrated the importance of knowing as much about the patient's background as possible, in order to allow the therapist to be able to successfully interpret the often confused information which the patient communicates. Because the patient's ability to express him/herself is often impaired by the dementing process, it is necessary for the therapist to be able to make accurate inferences about the meaning which the patient is attempting to convey. As was demonstrated in Sara's case history, past events are often merged with the present in a confusing and sometimes psychotically distorted manner, making interpretation extremely difficult for the uninformed caregiver. Since cognitive impairment interacts intimately with the personality and character of the individual, it is incumbent upon the caregiver to learn as much about this aspect of the patient as possible.

The techniques for learning about the patient are similar to those psychiatric interventions used for intact patients. It is most important to encourage the patient him/herself to speak about his/her past and to tell his/her story from his/her own perspective. All too often, the histories which are obtained about cognitively impaired individuals are derived solely from secondary sources because of the difficulty which these patients have with communication. As Peter Gay has observed, it is extremely difficult to write an accurate biography (Gay, 1988). Indeed, Freud himself, despite his historical approach to understanding, once commented "... biographical truth is not to be had, and even if one had it one could not use it." (Gay, 1988, p. XV). These observations highlight the importance of obtaining information directly from the patient, thereby allowing the therapist to experience some of the patient's emotional intensity, aroused when remembering the events of his/her life. Whether the events and the memories actually occurred is less critical than the fact that they have taken on meaning and reality for the patient and now form the basis for his/her thought content and emotional response.

Despite Freud's comments, it is self evident that an accurate and "factual" history can be obtained, and for this purpose ancillary, secondary sources may be crucial. Gene Cohen, in his chapter, has highlighted the importance of innovative approaches to history taking, such as audio and video recordings and the construction of a personal record for the patient. Additional techniques for enhancing the cargiver's awareness of the patient are the use of family albums, films and pictures which are reviewed both with the patient and the family. It is through these mechanisms that the patient's development and personality are reified and permit others to develop a deeper empathic understanding of the patient's current emotional life and inner self.

In taking a patient's history, it is important to connect their past life story with their present circumstances and behaviour. Understanding is derived from information about the patient's relationships, and most importantly their capacity to deal with the loss of these relationships and negotiate the vicissitudes of grief. Therapists should not give up the perspective of formulating a patient's current problem in the context of their past. The patient's personality characteristics, which began early in life, continue into old age. The basic strengths and weaknesses inherent in that development will still be evident in spite of the presence of cognitive impairment. For example, a patient's narcissistic need for admiration, which may be aggravating to staff, may be the most important element in the patient's self-esteem regulating mechanism. Behind the veil of their illness, such individuals may appear incompetent, unattractive and demanding, characteristics which often lead caregivers to wonder "who does she think she is?" when such patients boastfully demand admiration. The mode of expression of these narcissistic needs may be even more difficult to tolerate when patients express their narcissistic uncertainty, vulnerability and humiliation by "putting down" others. This type of behaviour is generally understandable particularly when there is a history of early life traumata and loss. It is constructive to see such behaviour as defensive and then to attempt to help the patient meet their needs in more appropriate ways.

Communication Diagnosis

Just as one makes a diagnosis of the illness process, so it is important to actively diagnose the communication capacity of the patient and then decide upon an appropriate level of psychotherapeutic intervention. As already noted, the first task is to gather information about the patient in order to develop a base of understanding. Thereafter, the therapist should determine, as carefully as possible, the patient's level of understanding, their memory resources, and their ability to orient themselves. Frequently, patients have difficulty comprehending verbal input, sometimes because of receptive problems and sometimes because of other factors such as high levels of anxiety or fear. As already noted, memory may be confused and disjointed because of disruptions in the patient's ability to construct an accurate time sequence. Similarly their ability to understand the meaning of environmental events may be impaired and orientation in space and time altered, leading the patient to feel constantly uncertain and insecure.

The patient's level of tolerance for interaction should be evaluated. Sometimes psychological testing is helpful and formal ADL assessment can also provide useful clues. The caregiver may look for evidence of anxiety and tension as the demands on the patient gradually become more complex. Some patients crave, and constantly seek, the companionship and reassurance of others. Other patients withdraw and cannot tolerate contact. One reclusive man for example, when asked to write a sentence as part of the mental status exam, wrote "When are you going to leave," thereby reinforcing the clear and consistent message he had always given to caregivers. He did not need or want the help of others.

Related to the assessment of tolerance is an awareness that the patient's capacity to do, to think, to understand and to communicate may fluctuate dramatically. Sometimes for example, there is a diurnal variation in the patient's abilities like sundowning, when the patient's cognitive state declines at night. Other factors such as fatigue, noise and confusion, or sensory deprivation, may make it unpredictably difficult for the patient to communicate at certain times, while at others it is much easier.

The communication diagnosis should include looking for specific stressors that interfere with the patient's ability to communicate. For example, the patient may have circumscribed paranoid fears of a roommate, or of a staff member which causes them to become highly anxious and withdrawn.

Finally, it is helpful to try and understand whether the patient's actions or statements have meanings which are not immediately obvious.

The agitated, cognitively impaired patient will often revert to stereotyped sounds, words, actions or movements when under stress. At other
times, the inner distorted, and sometimes psychotic, thought processes are
expressed in bizarre ways. For example, a moderately cognitively impaired
patient began to put spoonfuls of food on her sofa. No one quite
understood what was going on, until she began to speak about her daughter
who had died some years earlier. In her somewhat rambling, disjointed
way, she gradually revealed her belief that her daughter was lying on the
sofa, in a two-dimensional form. It was a poignant moment when we
realized that she believed she was feeding her daughter and that the food
went onto the couch because her daughter did not have any substance to her
head. With this context of understanding, obtained only by listening
carefully to the patient, her actions were not only comprehensible, but
permitted the staff to respond in a very specific, empathic and helpful
manner, to assist the patient in coping with her grief.

Capacity for Soothing

In assessing the patient's capacity to utilize different types of
psychotherapy, one important component is to evaluate his/her capacity
for soothing. As was evident in the case of Sara, some patients are able
to respond to personal contact and verbal intervention, while others are
not. The therapist should assess whether the patient is calmed by verbal
contact or more agitated by it? Does the patient demonstrate pleasure
when talking to others or is he/she merely agitated or withdrawn on
contact. Does he/she seem to seek out others? The therapist should
assess whether there is any sense of continuity between one session and
the next. Because of the inherent memory difficulties of cognitive
impairment, continuity and the soothing security it offers is often
apparently lost. Therapists should keep in mind however, that learning
does not cease entirely with impairment, but rather is slowed down
requiring much more repetition and practice. Frequent contact with the
patient may improve continuity. Finally the therapist should look for a
past history of soothing and relatedness in interpersonal relationships as
a clue to the patient's current capacity to utilize psychotherapeutic
interventions.

TECHNIQUES OF INTERVENTION

Whatever formal technical approach to therapy is employed, it will be
most effective if accompanied by accurate empathic rapport with the
patient. Empathic rapport and meaningful communication with others is a
basic human need. Cognitive impairment, particularly progressive
dementing illness, gradually erodes the resources necessary to establish

intimate, empathically rewarding relationships. The self-esteem and feelings of security of the patient are damaged because they may be unable to remember their past life, achievements and sources of support; they cannot mobilize their sources of support often because they are institutionalized and cut-off from others; and finally the progressive course of the illness, by its very nature, gradually impedes their capacity to relate and make themselves understood. It becomes the caregiver's responsibility to make clear to the patient that their needs for understanding and empathy are being attended to. Practical approaches may be on a very concrete and basic level. For example, a patient no longer able to comprehend what they read may respond to a comment such as - you must wish you could still read. Followed by - perhaps we can get someone to read to you. In other words, while an empathic statement of the caregiver's awareness of the patient's loss, in itself, is most important, it is further reinforced by a practical, concrete response to a problem that a patient may be having. However, caregivers should not feel that they must always try to meet the needs of their patients in a concrete manner. Frequently, simply conveying a sense of understanding, and providing the patient with a responsive listening ear, is the most crucial element in developing empathic rapport.

Psychotherapy for the cognitively impaired can be carried out either on an individual or group basis. Psychodynamically oriented group therapy has been successful with such individuals, although clearly, the modes of intervention must be titrated to the specific needs of the group. Groups may be led by a single therapist or by co-therapists.

Often, reminiscence is an early bridge between the members of the group, who may find it threatening to speak about their current situations. They seem much more able to expose their past lives, periods when they felt more intact and competent. Patients should be gradually encouraged to introduce their own emotionally important topics of discussion. The therapist should be active and facilitating, but temper the group's need for structure with an awareness of when to allow the group to find its own path.

The early life of such groups is often slow in its evolution, but, as indicated earlier in this chapter, experience suggests that these patients have a capacity to relate to each other and to develop a therapeutic rapport. This process is further facilitated if the therapist focuses on emotional process, not just concrete content. Using this approach, it is often possible to begin to look at issues of resistance, defensiveness, transference and countertransference, thereby deepening the level of discussion. Of course, one must be realistic about how far the patient's are able to proceed along such an abstract path of therapy. More severely impaired patients will have much greater difficulty and will often be entirely unable to engage in this form of treatment. However, many other patients, despite the presence of some cognitive impairment, welcome the depth and intensity of such group discussions. The themes which therapists can expect include loneliness, missed spouses, sexual attraction, faithfulness of partners, illness and fear of death, ward interactions, roommates and caregivers.

In both individual and group therapy, reminiscing is a universal process. It appears to improve self-cohesion and the maintenance of self-esteem, but as noted above, therapists must be cautious about mobilizing early unresolved conflicts which the patient has not got the ego strength to manage.

While psychotherapy is a verbal modality, the cognitively impaired patient often has difficulty with comprehension and expression of verbal content. Hence, non-verbal techniques are often a necessary adjunct and, for the more severely impaired, they become the major interactive modality. Various types of groups will be helpful in establishing communication with patients in the non-verbal mode. These include exercise groups, music, dance and movement groups, and various creative group activities. These groups should be viewed, not only as "activities" but also as interactive modes, whereby the therapist and other caregivers are able to derive a deeper understanding of the patients as well as providing the patient with vehicles of communication. Such groups reduce the sense of isolation often associated with cognitive decline and may *further* serve to enhance self-cohesion and self-esteem.

In instituting therapeutic modalities, therapists are well advised to avoid stereotyped "rules" and to attempt to adapt technique to the patient's need. For example, it has often been stated that the frail elderly require touching, sitting close and a loud voice. However, it is my experience that such individuals show a range of tolerance for this kind of intimate involvement. Hence, therapists should recognize the importance of evaluating the patient's need for touching and their requirements for personal space. While some patients miss the intimacy of touch and close involvement, others may be resentful or even panicked by such intimacy and intrusion. For example some demented patients seem to have a circle of inviolable personal space, and will aggressively strike out if others invade it without warning. Similarly the use of familiarity such as first names should be employed judiciously. Such approaches may be experienced as disrespectful, demeaning and aggressive or conversely, comforting depending on the needs of the patient, but it is the needs of the patient which must be determined first.

One difficult technical issue in therapy, either group or individual, is the question of reality orientation of the cognitively impaired.

As was evident in the case of Sara A., patients' communication is often illogical, unrealistic and accompanied by emotions which may be difficult to interpret. Under these circumstances the therapist must make a decision about how to intervene. The basic question is whether to correct the patient's reality, and if so, how to do it. Some patients are able to accept and allow such interventions and are able to borrow the staff's reality testing. In other circumstances, as was the case with Sara, correction of the patient may lead to feelings of rejection or humiliation, causing the patient to feel he/she is not believed. Correction of the patient's reality therefore, should be undertaken only after knowledge of the patient's sensitivities is gained.

Correction is especially difficult when the patient holds delusional beliefs. Delusions, in general, cannot be corrected by orientation-type feedback. The first step in responding is to make every effort to understand the nature of the delusion. For example, is it induced by environmental stimulation, leading to misinterpretation? An example comes from the case of a woman who routinely awoke during the night and screamed in terror because she believed there were snakes in her room. With careful questioning and evaluation, it became evident that she was reacting to the black plastic strip which bordered the wall of her room. The simple measure of providing her with adequate light and reassuring corrective feedback in the middle of the night calmed her fears and enabled her to get back to sleep. When delusions are environmentally based, it is important to keep the patient's environment as predictable, structured and simple as possible. Delusions must also be carefully evaluated for the "kernel of truth" which may reside within them. It is crucial that the therapists and caregivers be certain of their data and not attribute everything to the patient's disease and distortion.

Commonly, patients will develop entrenched delusions which become chronic and often are accompanied by severe agitation. For example, an institutionalized patient, who does not see family often enough, will sometimes begin to believe that a spouse, child or grandchild is dead or threatened, as in the case of Sara. The subsequent agitation may be handled in different ways. As Dr. Cohen has suggested, redirection may be a useful technique, prompting the patient to remember other areas of importance in their life and temporarily relinquishing the focus on the delusional belief. Some patients may have the capacity, with clues and memory aids, to remember the visit or phone call of the missing child, spouse, etc. Redirecting attention towards those events can be helpful in temporarily ameliorating the patient's anxiety. Gentle correction of reality, coupled with an empathic awareness of the patient's pain can also be calming. For example, one may say "it feels like people are dead when you don't see them enough. Your daughter is away on vacation, but she will return. I know you can't help but feel that she is gone forever".

Additional use of pictures and artifacts will also be helpful in prompting memory and in reinforcing a feeling of security and continuity within the patient. Finally, simple distraction, as one would use with a small child, can be helpful. For example, encouraging a patient to go for a walk or engage in a simple activity may be sufficient to redirect them away from the agitation of their delusion. Often, in spite of all these techniques, the overwhelming anxiety associated with reality distortions in cognitive impairment may require the use of medication as an adjunct to all the psychotherapeutic and environmental interventions. When necessary, these should not be avoided, since they make the patient much more accessible to all other interpersonal techniques of intervention.

Despite the fact that the patient's verbal expressions are of a delusional nature, it is often helpful to encourage the patient to verbalize their fears and anxieties. If this technique is to be used, it is important for a consistent caregiver to act as therapist and to set aside uninterrupted time which is guarded for the patient. It is important to be punctual since these patients require structure and predictability from caregivers as the basis for their communication. Their world is already unpredictable and confusing, hence the therapeutic intervention must supply counteracting elements.

Individual Therapy

Recognizing that the patients suffering from cognitive impairment will have varying capacities for, and receptiveness to, individual psycho-therapy, the therapist must be prepared to be flexible and to utilize a variety of approaches, some of which differ substantially from therapy with the cognitively intact patient. However, in spite of the difficulties, individual approaches can be very useful, both for understanding the patient, as well as developing methods of intervention which will help the patient cope with his/her evolving illness. Some of the basic techniques of individual therapy have been already discussed including the necessity for establishing an accurate empathic rapport, making a full communication diagnosis, and collecting complete data both from the patient and from ancillary sources. Once these steps are completed, it is then possible for the therapist to decide on the level of the patient's tolerance and the frequency of the contact. With the less intact cognitively impaired patient, it is useful to establish a pattern of frequent brief contacts ie., several times a week for 5-10 minutes. This kind of repetitive, consistent contact can facilitate the patient beginning to remember the therapist and the basic meaning of the sessions. For this group of patients, these brief contacts should stress concrete discussions.

The more impaired the patient, the less is his capacity to respond to abstract questions. Questions and comments which are short and require specific, brief answers from the patient are best. Open-ended questions can be confusing and agitating to patients who either may not comprehend the question, or are unable to gather the thoughts necessary for adequate expressive response. Similarly, the time frame of the patient's memory should be respected. Patients should not be pushed too hard to remember events which occurred outside their memory capacity since the patient will not be able to relate to them, and may become disturbed by his/her incapacity.

Cognitively impaired individuals are often very sensitive to non-verbal communication, such as tone of voice or body posture. A caregiver who addresses the patient over her/his shoulder while walking out of the room for example, or uses a patronizing tone unwittingly, may agitate the patient and lead to a breakdown of empathic rapport.

While therapy should not be frustrating, a balance must be struck with the patient, because it is important not to do for the patient what they are able to do for themselves. This applies not only to activities of daily living, but also to verbal interaction. When the patient is truly unable to provide answers or find the right word, then it can be helpful for the therapist to aid the patient. However, the therapist should wait until the patient has had a chance to verbalize his sometimes slow thinking process, and come up with an answer. As the therapist comes to know the patient more thoroughly, he/she will be able to understand when interventions and support are necessary and when the patient should be allowed to struggle.

Therapist Characteristics

Not every individual has either the interest or the training to engage cognitively impaired individuals in a psychotherapeutic activity, whether on an individual or group basis. Certain aspects of the therapist's personality and therapeutic skill will promote a more successful approach to treatment.

The therapist must be prepared for and able to tolerate the patient's often unfocused thoughts and statements, which at first sight may not make obvious sense. As we have tried to point out above, the patient's thoughts generally have a basis either in the stimulation of the immediate environment or arising from earlier memories. It is an important therapeutic capacity to be able to listen to the patient and to maintain an inquiring and interested stance toward what the patient says. Despite the repetitive nature of some patients' thoughts, the therapist will be most helpful if he is able to accept these repetitions as necessary to the patient's emotional well-being and as a manifestation of their helplessness to behave otherwise, in the face of their illness.

Because it is often necessary and important for debilitated and impaired individuals to be able to idealize the therapist, it is an important quality for the therapist to be able to accept this position vis-a-vis the patient. Sometimes, the unrealistic view of the patient can lead to uncomfortable feelings within the therapist because of his/her own knowledge of his/her own limitations. In contrast to work with younger or more intact individuals, this idealization may be most therapeutic if it is left unchallenged, unless it becomes necessary for the reality to be interpreted.

The flip-side of the coin of idealization is devaluation and rejection. Cognitively impaired individuals often resort to more primitive defenses, as indicated above. Their need to support their own threatened narcissism is often demonstrated by their attempts to devalue, and sometimes revile, their caregivers. The successful psychotherapist will be able to understand the nature of this process and both accurately interpret it, as well as accept the inevitability of it, in the context of the patient's need for this type of defensive structure.

Work with the impaired elderly is often a lonely activity, poorly understood and often not valued by colleagues. The therapist, therefore, must have the capacity to tolerate some therapeutic isolation. The isolation is further heightened by the fact that, in contrast to younger patients, the patient him/herself is often unable to offer the therapist the benefit of his own empathy, gratitude and caring. On the contrary, perhaps the most difficult element of this work lies in the responsibility of the therapist for maintaining and supporting so much of the therapeutic alliance, the continuity of the sessions and the interpretation of the material. He/she must remember the content of previous sessions and trigger the patient's memory actively by remembering for them.

Finally, recognizing the crucial nature of empathic relatedness, the therapist must have the capacity to both attempt to experience the patient's inner reality, while at the same time not being overwhelmed by feelings of hopelessness, fear and perhaps desperation. While it is necessary to be aware of the patient's losses and of the inner pain and turmoil with which they are struggling, the therapist must also be able to maintain an appropriate distance, in order to aid the patient and not be overwhelmed by the magnitude of their problems. A capacity to maintain realistic hopefulness is essential, but the therapist should guard against unrealistic expectations.

CONCLUSIONS

The cognitively impaired elderly, whether in institutions or living in the community, constitute a heterogeneous population with varying capacities and degrees of disability. In the early stages of decline, such individuals retain their basic personality and intellectual characteristics often remaining open and available to a wide range of psychotherapeutic approaches that require little modification. With advancing deterioration however, the capacity of the individual to fully participate in therapeutic processes gradually erodes placing an increasing burden on caregivers and therapists to define the nature of the problems and devise appropriate interventions, often without the awareness or cooperation of the patient him/herself.

Despite the difficulties which abound in dealing with the cognitively impaired, the literature, as a whole, clearly demonstrates that caregivers and therapists need not despair of being able to touch the remaining humanity in their patients. Recognizing that generalities may present a variety of pitfalls, and that each treatment activity must be specifically tailored to the needs of the individual patient, certain principles of therapy may be stated which can form the basis not only of treatment plans but also of future research.

The learning and behaviour techniques have proved often effective in the management of specific behaviours. However, the duration of their effect appears to be enhanced when behavioural approaches are incorporated in an on-going fashion as part of a global treatment program that incorporates milieu activity and educational approaches. In institutional settings, it is common for consultants to provide opinions about the management of specific problems, set-up programs, leave recommendations and retire from the scene. In chronic care institutions however, such interventions often lead to short-lived results, with units gradually reverting back to old patterns under the pressures of the day-to-day problems of caregiving. While brief intermittent intervention is possibly more cost effective, it is a worthwhile research question to ask whether long-term care institutions need a permanent team model of behavioural management rather than an intermittent consultative model.

The talking therapies, whether individual or group reveal the capacity of the cognitively impaired patient to respond to interactive, inter-personal techniques which maximize their sense of self and minimize feelings of fragmentation that result from the erosion of their cognitive capacities.

It is clear from the literature and from clinical experience that psychotherapeutic approaches to the cognitively impaired elderly can be rewarding for the therapist and often essential to the well-being of the patients. A variety of technical approaches are possible but one central feature of all therapies appears to be the presence of consistent, caring and empathic relationships, which are the basis for the successful implementation of most therapeutic programs. While group and milieu therapies have been the most commonly utilized modalities for this patient population, there is strong evidence that patients can be approached on an individual, psychotherapeutic basis using psychodynamic principles to inform therapy. However, a variety of techniques may be employed which are different from those used with younger patients. Finally, one must keep in mind that the work is arduous and that certain therapist characteristics are important components of the treatment process. Despite the fact that one is often dealing with an inexorable progressive illness with gradual decline and accompanying loss of capacity for relatedness and interaction, therapists and the therapeutic environment which they construct will work optimally if psychotherapeutic approaches and principles are incorporated into the overall process of therapy.

REFERENCES

Akerlund B.M., Norberg A. (1986). Group Psychotherapy with Demented Patients. Geriatric Nursing, 7, 83-84.

Allen K.S. (1976). A Group Experience for Elderly Patients with Organic Brain Syndrome. Health and Social Work, 1, 62-69.

Aronson M.K., Levin G., Lipkowitz R. (1984). A Community-Based Family/Patient Group Program for Alzheimer's Disease. Practice Concepts, 24, 339-342.

Barnes R.F., Raskind M.A., Scott M., Murphy C. (1981). Problems of Families Caring for Alzheimer Patients: Use of a Support Group. J. Am. Geriatr. Soc., 29, 80-85.

Berger L.F. (1978). Activating a Psychogeriatric Group. Psychiatr. Q., 50, 63-66.

Book H.E., Sadavoy J., Silver D. (1978). Staff countertransference to borderline patients on an inpatient unit. Am. J. of Psychother., 32, 521-532.

Brane, G. (1986). Normal Aging and Dementia Disorders - Coping and Crisis in the Family. Prog. Neuropsychopharmacol. Biol. Psychiatry, 10, 287-295.

Brody E., Kleban M.H., Lawton M.P., Silverman H.A. (1971). Excess Disabilities of Mentally Impaired Aged: Impact of Individualized Treatment. Gerontologist, 124-133, Summer, Part I.

Brody E.M., Kleban M.H., Lawton M.P., Moss M. (1974). Longitudinal Look at Excess Disabilities in the Mentally Impaired Aged. J. Gerontol., 29, 79-84.

Brook P., Degun G., Mather M. (1975). Reality Orientation, A Therapy for Psychogeriatric Patients: A Controlled Study. Br. J. Psychiatry, 127, 42-5.

Buckholdt D.R., Gubrium J.F. (1983). Therapeutic Pretense in Reality Orientation. Intl. J. Aging Hum. Dev., 16, 167-181.

Bulter, R. (1963). The life review: an interpretation of reminiscence in the aged. Psychiatry, 26, 65-76.

Cameron D.E. (1941). Studies in Senile Nocturnal Delirium. Psychiat. Q., 15, 47-53.

Charatan F.B. (1980). Therapeutic Supports for the Patient with OBS. Geriatrics, 35, 100-102.

Citrin R.S., Dixon D.N. (1977). Reality Orientation. A Milieu Therapy Used in an Institution for the Aged. Gerontologist, 17, 19-43.

Cosin L.Z., Mort M., Post F., Westrop C., Williams M. (1958). Experimental Treatment of Persistent Senile Confusion. Int. J. Soc. Psychiatry, 4, 24-42.

Cox K.G. (1985). Milieu Therapy. Geriatric Nursing. 6, 152-154.

Eisdorfer C., Cohen D. (1981). Management of the Patient and Family Coping with Dementing Illness. J. Fam. Pract., 12, 831-839.

Gay, P. (1988). Freud: A Life For Our Time. New York: W.W. Morton and Co.

Goldfarb A.I. (1967). Psychiatry in Geriatrics. Med. Clin. North Am., 51, 1515-1527.

Goldfarb, A.I., Sheps, J. (1954). Psychotherapy of the aged. Psychosom. Med., 16, 209-219.

Goldfarb A.I., Turner H. (1953). Psychotherapy of Aged Persons. II. Utilization and Effectiveness of "Brief" Therapy. Am. J. Psychiatry, 109, 916-921.

Gottesman L.E., Quarterman C.E., Cohn G.M. (1973). Psychosocial Treatment of the Aged. The Psychology of Adult Development and Aging. American Psychological Association, Washington.

Gwyther L.P., Blazer D.G. (1984). Family Therapy and the Dementia Patient. Am. Fam. Physician, 29, 149-156.

Haley W.E. (1983). A Family-Behavioral Approach to the Treatment of the Cognitively Impaired Elderly. Gerontologist, 23, 18-20.

Hanley I.G., McGuire R.J., Boyd W.D. (1981). Reality Orientation and Dementia: A Controlled Trial of Two Approaches. Brit. J. Psychiatry, 138, 10-14.

Harris C.S., Ivory P. (1976). An Outcome Evaluation of Reality Orientation Therapy with Geriatric Patients in a State Mental Hospital. Gerontologist, 16, 496.

Harris S., Snyder B., Snyder R., Magraw B. (1977). Behaviour Modification Therapy with Elderly Demented Patients: Implemen- tation and Ethical Considerations. J. Chronic Dis., 30, 129-134.

Holden U.P., Sinebruchow A. (1978). Reality Orientation Therapy: A Study Investigating the Value of this Therapy in the Rehabilitation of Elderly People. Age Ageing, 7, 83-90.

Hussian R.A. (1984). Behavioral Geriatrics. Progress in Behaviour Modification, Academic Press, Vol. 16, 159-183.

Kahn R.S. (1965). Comments - In Proceedings of the York House Institute on the Mentally Impaired Aged. Philadelphia: Philadelphia Geriatric Center.

Katz M.M. (1976). Behavioral Change in the Chronicity Pattern of Dementia in the Institutional Geriatric Resident. J. Amer. Geriatr. Soc., 24, 522-28.

LaVorgna D. (1979). Group Treatment for Wives of Patients with Alzheimer's Disease. Social Work in Health Care. 5, 219-221.

Lawton M.P. (1975). Geropsychological Knowledge as a Background for Psychotherapy with Older People. Presented at Symposium on Psychotherapy with the Aged. Annual Meeting of the American Psychological Association, Chicago, Illinois, September.

Lazarus L.W. (1976). A Program for the Elderly at a Private Psychiatric Hospital. Gerontologist, 16, 125-131.

Lazarus L.W. (1980). Self-Psychology and Psychotherapy with the Elderly: Theory and Practice. J. Geriatr. Psychiatry, 13, 69-88.

Lazarus L.W., Stafford B., Cooper K., Cohler B., Dysken M. (1981). A Pilot Study of an Alzheimer Patients' Relatives Discussion Group. Gerontologist, 21, 353-358.

Lazarus L.W., Weinberg J. (1982). Psychosocial Intervention with the Aged. Psychiatr. Clin. North Am., 5, 215-227.

Lazarus L.W., Cohler B.J., Lesser J. Self Psychology and the Late Life Dementias: Clinical Applications, Pre-publication manuscript.

Leng N. (1982). Behavioural Treatment of the Elderly. Age Ageing, 11, 235-243.

Lesser J., Lazarus L.W., Frankel R., Havasy S. (1981). Reminiscence Group Therapy with Psychotic Geriatric Inpatients. Gerontologist, 21, 291-296.

Levine N.B., Dastoor D.P., Gendron C. (1983). Coping with Dementia. J. Amer. Geriatr. Soc., 31, 12-17.

Levine N.B., Gendron C., Dastoor D.P. et al (1984). Existential Issues in the Management of the Demented Elderly Patient. Am. J. of Psychother., 38, 215-223.

Linden M. (1953). Group Psychotherapy with Institutionalized Senile Women. Studies in Gerontologic Human Relations. Int. J. Group Psychother., 3, 150-170.

Linden M. (1957). The Promise of Therapy in the Emotional Problems of Ageing. Paper delivered at the Fourth Congress of International Association of Gerontology. Merano, Italy.

Manaster A. (1972). Therapy with the "Senile" Geriatric Patient. Int. J. Group Psychother., 22, 250-257.

Mann S.H. (1986). Practical Management Strategies for Families with Demented Victims. Neurol. Clin., 4, 469-477.

McEvoy C.L., Patterson R.L. (1986). Behavioural Treatment of Deficit Skills in Dementia Patients. Gerontologist, 26, 475-478.

Merriam S. (1980). The Concept and Function of Reminiscence: A review of the research. Gerontologist, 20, 604-609.

Miller E. (1977). The Management of Dementia: A Review of Some Possibilities. Br. J. Soc. Clin. Psychol., 16, 77-83.

Pollock D.D., Liberman R.P. (1974). Behavior Therapy of Incontinence in Demented Inpatients. Gerontologist, 14, 488-491.

Ratna L., Davis J. (1984). Family Therapy with the Elderly Mentally Ill. Some Strategies and Techniques. Br. J. Psychiatry, 145, 311-315.

Reichenfeld H.F., Czapo K., Carmire L., Gardner R. (1973). Activity Programs on a Geriatric Ward.

Roskos S.R., Lerner S., Kline, B.E. (1979). The Elderly Patient in a Therapeutic Community. Comprehensive Psychiatry, 20, 359-369.

Sadavoy J. (1987). Character Disorders in the Elderly: An Overview. In Sadavoy. J, Leszcz, M. (ed.). Treating the Elderly with Psychotherapy. Madison, Ct.: International Universities Press. 175-229.

Schafer S.C. (1985). Modifying the Environment. Geriatric Nursing, 6, 157-159.

Schmidt, G.L., Keyes, B. (1985). Group psychotherapy with family cargivers of demented patients. Gerontologist, 25, 347-350.

Schwab M., Rader J., Doan J. (1985). Relieving the Anxiety and Fear in Dementia. J. Gerontological Nursing, 11, 8-15.

Silver A. (1950). Group Psychotherapy with Senile Psychotic Patients. Geriatrics, 5, 147-150.

Steuer J. (1982). Psychotherapy with the Elderly. Psychiat. Clin. North Am., 5, 199-213.

Teusink, J.P, Mahler S. (1984). Helping Families Cope with Alzheimer's Disease. Hospital and Community Psychiatry, 35, 152-156.

Whyte C.R., Constantopoulos C., Bevans H.G. (1982). Types of Countertransference Identified by Q-Analysis. British Psycholog. Soc., 55, 187-201.

Wisner E., Green M. (1986). Treatment of a Demented Patients Anger with Cognitive Behavioural Strategies. Psychological Reports, 2, Part I, 447-450.

Yalom I.D, Terrazas F. (1968). Group Therapy for Psychotic Elderly Patients. Am. J. Nurs., 68, 104-112.

CHAPTER 6

HELPING THE FAMILY

Graham Berman, M.B., Ch.B., F.R.C.P.(C)
Baycrest Centre for Geriatric Care
University of Toronto
Toronto, Ontario

Optimal treatment of the elderly patient with brain disorder usually demands close involvement of the family. The emotional well-being of the patient is intertwined with that of the family. And the practical tasks of everyday life with the patient often require profound changes in the way the family functions.

Personal relationships are central to most of our activities. Personality is formed, satisfactions achieved, and lives lived out in interaction with important others. The social context will determine the emotional and practical fate of our brain-disordered patients and their families.

THE SOCIAL NETWORK

Each person occupies a place in a social network. The network can be conceptualized as an array of interactive interdependent individuals, in which the degree of emotional and instrumental interdependence of any pair is an inverse function of their distance from each other. Members of each nuclear family will be closely connected. A change in one member will have important effects on all of them. At an increased distance in the array will be members of the extended family, and close friends. There will be other social, work-connected, and recreation-connected relationships, marginally affecting and affected by changes in the nuclear family, but more likely to move out of the proximal network if a change in the nuclear family removes the original function of the association. Chronic illness, then, may result in significant constriction in the social network of the patient and of the caretaker-partner.

The area I have discussed is the natural network, the set of mutual personal relationships. In addition to these, facultative connections may be made with the professional network, the more distal set of community functions, available to support those individuals and families whose adaptive systems require augmentation.

THE PROXIMAL NETWORK: THE FAMILY SYSTEM

The family structure constitutes a homeostatic system which controls and balances the actions of its members. Each nuclear family develops operational rules which determine its power and role structure, its modes of decision making in various areas, its methods of conflict resolution. Different topics will be dealt with in different ways. Some types of affective expression will be encouraged, others suppressed. The family develops monitoring and feedback systems by which any departure from the accepted range of behaviour is modulated. The family and its members are changing constantly, with the result that the operating system is being re-negotiated. Each change requires mutual readjustments among the members, with varying degrees of tension and instability in the system. Generally a larger family group will more easily absorb change, while a smaller group may be more severely disturbed by a change in one member. The two-person group of many older nuclear families in our mobile society will be relatively less resilient to change.

Outside the nuclear geriatric couple, but still part of the proximal network, are the families of the adult children of the couple. They are likely to be involved in their own nuclear families, but to some extent still caught up in the rules and needs of their families of origin. At times of stress in the original family the adult child may divert energy and participation from his or her newer family, to assist the parental unit. This may constitute a significant and damaging stress to the younger family. The conflict of loyalties to spouse and to parent constitutes a dilemma that some families do not satisfactorily resolve.

PROXIMAL NETWORK: ADAPTIVE SYSTEMS

The homeostatic family system buffers the effect of change. The family of a brain-disordered patient adopts a hierarchical series of buffering and compensatory strategies which depend on their previously established coping style and on the particular role which the patient held in the family.

A woman was suffering increasing memory impairment. She and her husband had been active, good-humoured, and quite flexible in their

family roles. As the illness developed they coped emotionally by
joking and laughing about her lapses, while in a practical way the
husband took over the tasks his wife could not manage. The practical
adaptation worked well. The affective coping style was consistent
with their previous social personalities, and demanded less
constriction of social relationships than often occurs, but left them
unsupported in their individual feelings of loss and of anxiety about
the future.

A man suffering a similar memory loss had always dominated his family,
demanding obedience and servitude. He and his wife were still
working. She assumed a number of his instrumental functions, while
retaining her diffident, submissive manner, in order to minimize
deviation from the family structure. If she became assertive in
manner, her husband would pull her back by an irritated gesture or
comment. To help cope with the unexpressed depression and the strain
of keeping up a normal appearance, the couple withdrew from all social
and recreational activities except watching television. Increasing
memory loss forced the patient to retire from work. His wife
continued to work for three hours a day. This represented such a
departure from his dominant role that he became increasingly irritable
with her, demanding more and more time and attention. She now sensed
an opportunity to rebel against the tyranny, and insisted despite his
anger that she would continue working. He developed the delusion that
she was having an affair with a co-worker. This was an escalation in
the power he was using to re-establish the family rules, and she was
sufficiently upset by it that she acceded. She retired, looked after
him, and his delusion was dropped. Again, the style of adaptation was
consistent with the previous mode of family functioning, and preserved
the role structure. Clearly, the adaptive efforts of the family may
seem counter-productive. Sometimes help towards change is accepted.
In the case discussed, outside interference was not, at that stage,
acceptable to the family.

When the functional impairment of the patient is so severe as to
render previous coping methods useless, major role changes may be forced
on the family. A partner who has never handled financial matters may have
to take over. Or one who has never assumed nurturing functions may now be
the principal caretaker of the patient. More often than not a healthy
partner adapts well to the new role, in part because the change has the
implicit support of the disabled spouse. When the marriage has been a
good one, the well member sometimes expresses great willingness to care
for the spouse out of a sense of love and affection and a wish to preserve
the reassuring and comforting life of the relationship.

As the stresses of the illness require more support than simply an adjustment in the couple system, or when the patient does not have a spouse, more responsibility is transferred to the extended family if it is available. The degree to which the adult children and their families have been involved in the parental family system is a determinant of the readiness with which they now become involved. The larger the group of people participating in the system, the more easily will adaptation occur. Usually, however, one person, either spouse or child, will be the primary caretaker. An important consideration, then, is whether the involvement of the adult child can be assimilated into his or her nuclear family system, or whether it becomes disruptive. When the second generation family is experiencing system difficulties there is a greater chance that the demands of the parental family will become disruptive. The needs of the parent may then be used as an external focus for the expression of those difficulties.

SPECIAL PROBLEMS OF THE PROXIMAL FAMILY

1. **The caretaker role:** The care of a chronically ill member of the family is an immense burden physically and emotionally. The small, usually 2-person, elderly family has little buffering capacity. The drastic role-changes and quite different way of life severely test the adaptive abilities of the caretaker.

At the same time, the quite sudden loss of the social network resulting from the more constricted life style, removes many of the rest and recreational activities and their attendant relationships.

2. **Mutual Depression:** Sadness about the loss of health, loss of a healthy partner, the loss of an experienced and hoped-for way of life, is almost inevitably a consequence of the illness in the patient and in the close family. Often there is nobody in the family who feels free to express or acknowledge the sadness. The caretaker feels he or she must boost the patient's spirits by remaining cheerful while the patient is afraid that to express sadness will alienate others. A somewhat artificial and mutually distancing atmosphere develops, and neither partner feels able to elicit a real sense of intimacy with the other. In fact, patient and caretaker are often capable of a real and valuable mutual expression of feeling, and feel greatly supported and valued when helped to share this support with each other.

In other families the capacity for such mutuality is lacking, either because it was never possible in the family, or because the illness is too severe. It is then important to acknowledge and discuss the sadness and sense of unfairness which the caretaker experiences.

3. **Need for Information and Support:** The complexities of the medical and social service systems are quite daunting to most people. Many patients and families need to do considerable questioning as they struggle to understand the nature of the illness, its prognosis, and the possibilities of successful treatment. Families often need to be able to explore alternative and unorthodox treatment modalities in their desperate search for a cure, but they must then feel free to return to the original medical service for treatment without fearing criticism for having explored other opinions.

Well-being of family and patient will depend on the development of a co-operative relationship between them and the treatment group. This requires that patient and relatives be treated with respect and concern, and that information about the treatment facilities, their limitations, and the alternatives be discussed with them in a way they can easily understand. Support groups and information groups may be a valuable adjunct.

4. **Caretaker Burnout:** The drastic change in responsibility, routine and activity, together with the loss of support from the ill partner and from the now constricted social network, constitute major stresses to the caretaker. The caretaker can be helped by a range of practical supportive measures from the extended family and from the professional network of social services. These include ongoing relief measures such as assistance with nursing care or meal preparations, and weekly relief periods which allow the caretaker a day off for recreation. They also include periodic vacations, when temporary home-care or hospitalization services allow the caretaker a longer recovery period. The supportive and recreational needs of caretakers vary immensely. Some have low tolerance for their roles despite what seems like relatively light instrumental burdens, while others withstand immense demands with great patience. It is important to adapt relief services to the needs of the caretaker, and not to confuse those needs with the condition of the patient, for these two variables are poorly correlated.

SPECIAL PROBLEMS OF THE PROFESSIONAL NETWORK

1. **Community Position Produces Conflict of Interests:** The professionals serving the elderly are often employed by a governmental or other bureaucratic organization rather than by the family of the patient. Support and treatment facilities are scarce relative to the demand, and the family usually lacks financial resources to purchase alternative services. The professional occupies the mediating position between the needy patient family and the restrictive bureaucracy of which he or she is an agent. It is sometimes difficult for the professional to avoid

identifying with the powerful institution in an attitude of arrogant rejection of the needs and anxieties of the family and patient. It is important, despite membership of the power group, to connect empathically with the client, to define clearly what might be in the best interests of the patient and family, and to discuss candidly without defensiveness, the facts of the situation and the limitations of the support and treatment facilities.

2. **Difficulty Understanding Limitations of the Elderly:** It is extraordinarily hard to identify with the rigid clinging to a familiar past and the terror of relinquishing any symbol of it, which characterizes many old people. As mental flexibility declines, adaptive functioning becomes increasingly dependent on the familiar context and associated routines. A move to new quarters, even to a different room, is frightening and disorganizing. Yet the organization of our institutions often necessitates discontinuities in care and context which render mental and physical changes even more frightening to patients and families.

3. **Difficulty Understanding Sadness of Loss:** One expects the elderly to become progressively disabled, and therefore tends to block empathic understanding of their intense sadness as capacities disappear and hopes are abandoned. The professional tends to ignore the sadness, and so fails to connect with the central experience of the aging family.

4. **Difficulty Recognizing the Competence of the Patient and Family:** The suppliers of services are aware of a range of possibilities, have limited time to spend with clients, and frequently fail to connect sufficiently with each family member, including the patient, to form a working alliance with the competent aspects of the patient and family. The result is that the family members, or the patient, feel patronized, and mistrustful of the decisions which are made.

ASSESSMENT OF PATIENT AND FAMILY

Assessment and treatment are co-operative undertakings between patient, family, and professionals. The purpose, nature and limitations of the inquiry should be explicit, and understood by all involved.

The following points might be included:

1. The nature of the patients disability:
    - how does the patient conceptualize it?
    - how does the main caretaker see it?
    - how do other members of the proximal network see it?
    - to what extent can differences in conceptualization be reconciled?

2. The remaining adaptive capability of the patient:
   - how does each person see it?
   - can differences in conceptualization be reconciled?
3. The role structure in the nuclear family:
   - how explicitly are roles defined?
   - is the structure similar to roles defined earlier in the
        family history?
   - if so, how have the roles been preserved?
   - if not, how and why have the roles changed?
4. The family's instrumental functioning:
   - how are practical tasks performed?
   - how much flexibility is apparent?
   - how much reserve capacity?
   - how much stress is apparent?
   - to what extent is extended family involved?
   - in what ways might community resources support or increase the
        capacity?
5. The family's affective functioning:
   - what affects are expressed, and by whom?
   - what affects are suppressed, and by whom?
   - when is affective expression used adaptively, supportively?
   - when is affective expression maladaptive and interfering with
        family function?
   - if maladaptive, or overly constricted, is there capacity for
        change?
6. How is the patient's disability incorporated into the family
   system?
   - is role definition a consequence of the illness?
   - if so, is this necessary and useful?
7. The feed-back mechanisms used to maintain the family system:
   - how adaptive are they?
   - if restricting adaptation, is there capacity for change?
8. The degree of change from earlier functioning of the family:
   - change in boundaries of the family group;
   - change in social network;
   - change in activities;
   - extent to which these are adaptive or maladaptive.
9. The boundaries of the family system:
   - to what extent are families of the patient's children
        involved?
   - to what extent are other parts of the family and the social
        network involved?
   - how adaptive are these involvements?
10. The effects on other parts of family group:
   - the capacity of children of the patient to help;

  - the stresses on the family of the children resulting from the
      changes;
  - the adaptive or maladaptive qualities of the involvement;
  - if maladaptive (e.g. a source of contention or stress in the
      second generation family) is capacity for change apparent?

TREATMENT OF THE FAMILY

Assessment will have outlined the adaptive strengths, the reserve
buffering capacities, and the areas of stress and difficulty in the
nuclear family and its proximal network.

Discussions with the family allow an estimate of the potential to use
various kinds of assistance. The whole range of therapeutic techniques
may be used, but most commonly, fairly simple supportive or strategic
methods are most valuable. The following are examples.

1. Explanation and Discussion

The therapist can help the family increase their adaptive potential by
using explanation and mutual discussion of relevant parts of the
diagnosis, assessment and treatment. It should be noted that the
assessment process, carried out in a relaxed, co-operative manner is, in
itself, valuable in setting before the family an outline of the factors
one might consider, of an objective attitude to these factors, and of a
practical orientation to their situation.

2. Reshaping Instrumental Functions

Instrumental functions may sometimes be improved by re-defining them
and shaping their practice. Often this may be achieved by simple
explanation and discussion. Sometimes, however, maladaptive instrumental
functioning is part of a wider set of system distortions, which are
important in the maintenance of, for example, an obsolete role structure.
The family will then resist change which represents to them the loss of a
vestige of the old family.

In one family the husband had always kept rigid control over all
expenditures. He had insisted that supermarket shopping be done when
he could be present, which was also during the most crowded period of
the shopping day. When his neurological disorder precluded his
accompanying his wife, he still demanded that she keep the same
inconvenient routine. In this and other ways he tried to deny the
disability. His wife co-operated, at considerable cost to her sense

of well-being, but fearing that to oppose him would distress him further. The man's illness was a further source of power in his interaction with his wife. The therapist structured a treatment schedule for the man which required his wife's presence during what had been the shopping hours. In this way the man seemed to be in control of the decision that his wife should now shop at a different time. The wife's new routine seemed to be subordinate to the man's needs, but in fact was arranged to be very much more convenient for her.

3.   Increased Affective Capacity

The ability of a couple to support each other can be increased by therapeutic work on their affective communication. The high prevalence of depression in patients and spouses is accompanied by constriction of affective interaction, with loss of supportive intimacy. Sensitive work on the interaction of the couple is useful in restoring a comforting closeness.

A therapist may help the couple to reminisce about their life together, about the illness and its effects, and to acknowledge the sadness from which they have tried to protect one another. They are surprised to find the sharing of feeling restores their intimacy and their ability to support each other.

Often the affective constriction has included a loss of sensual touching and sexual play. The loss of self-esteem flowing from the disability renders the patient afraid to ask for sensual closeness and the caretaker sometimes feels that to seek it is inappropriate. Neurological illness also tends to change the texture and resilience of the patient's body, interfering with the established system of signal and response. Simple sex therapy techniques, together with explanation, enable some couples to re-establish a valuable physical intimacy.

4.   Restructuring the Extended Family

The close relatives may become excessively involved in the instrumental functions of the patient and spouse, inducing unnecessary dependency. Therapeutic work with the family defines boundaries between the generations and encourages a better level of adaptive function in the patient.

5.   Prophylactic Restructuring of the Extended Family

The married child of the patient sometimes becomes so involved in the illness of the parent as to endanger his or her own family. This may occur when a spouse is intolerant of the disturbance, or it may serve as an external focus for conflict already present in the younger marriage. Various combinations of transgenerational treatment and marital therapy will define appropriate generational boundaries, and negotiate acceptable compromises between the younger spouses.

7. Self-Help Groups

The sense of isolation and uniqueness is disturbing to many families. Encouraging them to compare their experiences with those of others in similar situations and to talk of stresses and coping mechanisms, and to learn more about support services can be invaluable in helping them tolerate the stress of the illness and caretaking.

CONCLUDING COMMENT

The quality of life of the patient and family depend on their capacity to cope with the special stresses of their situation. Examination of the patient in the context of family and community allows a diagnosis of the particular sources of stress and the areas to which professional resources might most efficiently be directed to shore up adaptive capacity.

A wide variety of simple and practical therapeutic strategies are available to help the family augment their coping abilities.

CHAPTER 7

MANAGEMENT OF DISRUPTIVE BEHAVIOURS IN THE
COGNITIVELY IMPAIRED ELDERLY: INTEGRATING
NEUROPSYCHOLOGICAL AND BEHAVIOURAL APPROACHES

Guy-Bernard Proulx, Ph.D.
Baycrest Centre for Geriatric Care
Toronto, Ontario

Neuropsychology has experienced unprecedented growth in the last
ten years. Its focus has been almost exclusively on description and
diagnosis. Most of the literature in the field discusses how various
cognitive deficits relate to underlying neuropathologies. Little
attention has been given to treatment and management issues.

Rehabilitation and treatment of cognitive deficits is now being
addressed because of the increasing number of severe head injury survivors
and the recent impetus in the field of geriatrics and dementia. Authors
are only beginning to recognize how cognitive deficits interfere with
patients' psychosocial adjustments (Lezak, 1988). Barbara Wilson (1987)
recently commented that neurologically impaired people and their families
would benefit considerably if neuropsychology strengthened its links with
clinical psychology. Wilson believes that if the emphasis on intervention
strategies, normally practiced by the behaviourally-oriented clinical
psychologist, was shared with neuropsychology both disciplines would be
greatly enhanced. Because of social pressures, the field of cognitive
rehabilitation will most likely continue to expand and increase in
popularity over the coming years.

The new field of cognitive rehabilitation has been mostly geared
towards young victims of brain damage. Most head-injured youths and their
families are demanding services because of their need to maximize social
and vocational reintegration. George Prigatano (1986) in his book,
Neuropsychological Rehabilitation After Head Injury identifies three
levels of retraining as being most popular in cognitive rehabilitation.
The first is to help patients become aware of their residual cognitive
deficits. Deficits can be elicited, for example, in a supportive and
therapeutic environment to help patients become more familiar with their

147

limitations and to learn to readjust their expectations more realistically. The next approach is to teach patients methods of substitution and compensation using intact brain functions to bypass the deficits. A third approach is to train patients to improve underlying functional deficits. Many practitioners are pessimistic, however, regarding the benefits of directly treating cognitive disorders. Nevertheless, an increasing number of head-injured people spend the rest of their lives trying to "habilitate" or learn to make the best of their residual strengths after being discharged from hospital.

As it is currently practiced, cognitive rehabilitation is often impractical because of significant disruptive behaviours which develop as an overlay to underlying cognitive disorders. This is especially the case in geriatrics. When various dementias have been diagnosed and profiles of spared and impaired cognitive functions delineated, caregivers may be overwhelmed by the magnitude of psychosocial problems that result from brain damage. Other confounding issues complicating cognitive rehabilitation in the elderly are that cognitive deficits are frequently compounded by multiple chronic systemic illnesses and toxic effects of medications. In addition, a majority of demented patients are unaware of their cognitive deficits. Caregivers can benefit from learning more about specific cognitive disorders and how they translate into everyday behaviours. They need to understand how cognitive disorders interact with environmental factors to trigger disruptive behaviours. Careful attention to context and to the less readily observed cognitive deficits is essential for understanding, predicting and controlling behaviours that impede the patients' quality of life and that of the caregivers. A more pragmatic approach incorporating behaviour management techniques is needed, therefore, to help caregivers deal with the behavioural and social outcomes of cognitive deficits.

Hussian and Davis (1985) describe behaviour management as an attempt to change the frequency, intensity, duration or location of specific problem behaviours or sets of behaviours through systematically varying antecedent stimuli or consequential events. It is much broader in scope than the traditional classical or operant conditioning approaches. It incorporates social variables as well as cognitive variables that help improve patients' quality of life. Their model can be operationalized by what has become known as the ABC approach to behavioural analysis. It is based on the premise that behaviour is intertwined with environmental events immediately preceding and following the occurrence of the behaviour (Jackson and Patterson, 1982). The three components of the ABC model are:

Antecedent (A): The observable environmental event(s) or situation(s) occurring immediately before the observed targeted behaviour.

Behaviour (B): The observable targeted behavioural response of the patient. This could be a specific inappropriate behaviour that is interfering with the patient's quality of life. It could also be an appropriate behaviour that needs to be reinforced.

Consequence (C): The observable environmental event(s) or situation(s) occurring immediately after the observed behaviour. Often, this is the response of the caregiver to a specific behaviour from the patient.

The ABC model is extensively used by behaviour clinicians who work with children and younger adults. Unfortunately, a technical lag has occurred in its application to the cognitively-impaired elderly (Patterson, 1987). The following is the typical sequence of a behavioural management approach to patients with cognitive disorders:

1. A neuropsychological evaluation of cognitive deficits and strengths for use in the design of an individualized treatment program. A poor understanding of the cognitive disorders may lead to responses which exacerbate inappropriate behaviours.

2. A clear definition and identification of a specific behaviour targeted for management. A common error is to try and manage several behaviours at once.

3. Systematic observations of the specific targeted behaviour using ABC charting and other observational tools. Table 1 is an example of ABC charting.

4. Baseline measurements, of type, frequency and duration of the inappropriate behaviour are clearly charted so it is amenable for feedback to caregivers or to patients.

5. Design of a multi-dimensional treatment program for the management of the targeted behaviour. Treatment modalities may include neuro-psychological counselling with families and professional caregivers that helps them to readjust their demands and expectations according to the nature of the cognitive disorders. Other intervention strategies may include: basic training in how to reinforce or extinguish certain behaviours; introducing environmental changes that may help to compensate for some of the cognitive dysfunctions responsible for the disruptive behaviour; using classical psychotherapeutic interventions to maximize the adjustment of caregivers.

6. Implementation and coordination of the treatment program.

7. Evaluation, feedback and monitoring of the treatment program. Re-introduction of the protocol as a follow-up measure is useful to monitor progress and maintain the gains.

The following case studies illustrate controlled behavioural programs for the evaluation and management of disruptive behaviours in patients with severe cognitive disorders. Patients were given neuropsychological assessments to identify cognitive deficits and strengths for use in their treatment programs. Throughout the programs, data were continually collected to provide an objective means of determining the outcome of the treatment programs.

CASE 1 - Mr. T.B. *

Mr. T.B. was a 78-year-old man who showed increasingly abnormal behaviour over the course of 4 years. He had a history of memory loss and recently had displayed paranoid-like behaviours. In particular, he was preoccupied with things breaking and with his fear of strangers and of fire. He would, at times, strike himself on the head and throw stones at people passing in the street. Although he had paranoid ideation, there were no hallucinations. There was little indication of depression. Within the past year, he was admitted to a psychiatry ward of a local, acute-care hospital where he was treated with anti-psychotic medication. He was subsequently referred for a neurological evaluation. The EEG showed a mild focal slowing of activity bilaterally over the temporal lobes. The CT suggested a marked degree of cerebral atrophy and relatively large multiple infarctions of the left posterior temporal and right anterior and mid-temporal regions. The patient was subsequently transferred to a Geriatric Day Hospital and referred for a neuropsychological evaluation of his cognitive functioning.

The patient had no insight into his deficits. He was particularly disoriented for time. On simple tests of attention, he did quite well. He could, for example, repeat up to 5 numbers forward. When tasks were slightly more difficult and demanded more concentrated effort (such as counting by 3s or counting backwards), his performance deteriorated remarkably. The manner in which errors were made revealed a noteworthy pattern. Initially he did well, but he soon appeared to forget the "rules" of the task. He, therefore, clearly understood the instructions but could not retain the information.

*Portions of this case study appeared in Clinical Gerontologist, Vol. 6, No. 2, February, 1986, pp. 121-128.

This was apparent on all tests of verbal and non-verbal memory. Although he could register information (repetition, simple auditory comprehension), he could not retain any of the information even after a few seconds delay. He did well on tests of remote memory, but needed cues to assist him to retrieve the information. Language functions - repetition, auditory comprehension, reading and writing were relatively well-preserved but paraphasias, problems with naming and mild difficulties with praxis were observed. Tests of perceptual and constructional abilities were normal as were tests of stereognosis and finger tapping. It was concluded that he had severe anterograde amnesia and had great difficulty learning anything new, except by rote. These results were consistent with large, multiple bilateral infarctions of the temporal lobes.

Given his lasting disturbance of memory, disorientation, apathy and agitation, it was decided to place him on a behavioural management program in an attempt to alleviate his so-called paranoid tendencies. At home, his wife was asked to analyse problematic behaviours in terms of their relationships to other events. She was asked to keep a daily log of events antecedent to the inappropriate behaviour and her responses to the behaviour. The goal was to provide information about the frequency and the duration of the "paranoid-like" behaviours as well as the nature of the responses that maintained them. We suspected that many of these inappropriate behaviours were secondary to the severe cognitive deficits and exacerbated by particular triggers.

Behavioural Management Program

To obtain a meaningful and quantitative understanding of Mr. T.B.'s disorder, he was put on a controlled behavioural management program. Since he was an outpatient (coming to the Day Program only twice a week), his wife served as the "behavioural observer". She was supplied with an ABC chart and asked to indicate when the problematic behaviour occurred and to provide a description of the behaviour in as much detail as possible. Furthermore, she was asked to record precisely what events preceded and followed the behaviour. The first week of observation served as a "baseline" period. As such, no intervention was attempted. A sample of the first week's ABC is illustrated in Table 1. Over this baseline period, 30 "confused-paranoid" behaviours were noted. A number of features of the ABC chart were striking. First, his wife was able to report adequately the problematic behaviour and its antecedents. Unfortunately, she often neglected to report the responses to the behaviour in sufficient detail to allow precise analysis. Nevertheless, it was readily apparent that many of the behaviours, previously described as confused, occurred immediately upon awakening in the morning and after

TABLE 1: BASELINE OBSERVATION PERIOD

Date	Time	Antecedent Behaviour	Problem Behaviour	Consequential Behaviour
08-09	0800	Got up from sleep	"Where are my pants? Did you take my stuff away?"	Wife: "What stuff?" TB: "My money. I haven't a cent. You leave me broke. Come on. Give me my money.
28-09	1530	Got up from nap	"What goes up to the roof?" (Removes cobble stones). "The things are up to the ceiling."	Wife: "What things?" TB: "I don't know. There's a name for it. Come look it over. See the paper on the bed." Wife: "There isn't any paper.
02-10	0830	Had breakfast	"Do we go to school today?"	Wife: "You mean the Day Centre (at the hospital). TB: "Yes. Are there any kids here to go to school?"

naps. In still later ABC reports, it was noted that naps occurred at predictable times, after lunch, in the early afternoon.

Prinz and Raskind (1978) have observed that disorientation upon awakening is fairly common in the aged. Hachinski, Lassen and Marshall (1974) describe nocturnal confusion as being one of the clinical features of multiple infarct dementia. Excessive daytime sleepiness and resultant confusion may also be common in the elderly (Miles and Dement, 1985). Finally, daytime sleepiness has been found to fluctuate on an approximately 90 minute cycle (Broughton, 1975) and may well peak in the early afternoon during the so-called "post-lunch dip". This man's confusional state appeared to occur during periods of low arousal. It was also apparent that his wife was reinforcing the inappropriate behaviour. She often queried his confused and aphasic statements which consequently led to its continuation as he attempted to work through his already muddled flow of logic.

In the second and subsequent weeks, his wife was asked to provide even more details of her husband's behaviour patterns and to pay closer attention to her own reactions to the problem behaviour. She was told to ignore his confused behaviour as much as possible (not to respond to his "bizzare", inappropriate questions or if this were not possible to change the topic) and to reinforce appropriate behaviours. She was also encouraged to reduce the number of his daily naps. The number of confused and paranoid behaviours dropped to 20 in the second week (see Figure 1). At the end of the second week of monitoring, instructions were again provided regarding the need for reinforcing proper behaviours and ignoring of inappropriate behaviour. In the weeks that followed, the incidence of inappropriate behaviour leveled off at approximately 10 per week. These occurred mainly upon awakening in the morning. In these cases, T.B. was still unable to separate reality from unreality. The family reported that the reduction of daily naps almost eliminated periods of "nocturnal confusions" (confused, disoriented behaviour following awakenings during the night).

Discussion

While Mr. T.B.'s confusional-disoriented state was largely a result of his memory disorder and a poor understanding of his aphasic difficulties by his family, it was only after a precise behavioural assessment of his daily home situation that a consistent, antecedent triggering agent became apparent. Mr. T.B.'s "paranoid" state most often followed periods of sleep or naps. His wife, by responding with concern to his confused, disoriented aphasic questions, unwittingly led to their continuation by evoking further confusion and in all likelihood, subsequent exasperation. She was helped to understand that much of the bizzare speech and behaviour was in fact paraphasic language and post-awakening confusion. As she learned to withhold responding to these behaviours and to reinforce appropriate behaviours, they declined dramatically. The confused and paranoid-like behaviours reached a stable level occurring at quite predictable times.

CASE 2 - Mr. L.S.

Mr. L.S. was a 67-year-old man on a continuing care unit, who was referred to the Department of Psychology for management of disruptive behaviours. Staff found him to be demanding, noisy, agitated and uncooperative.

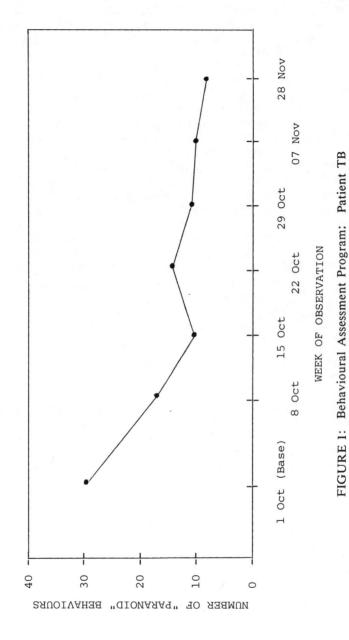

FIGURE 1:   Behavioural Assessment Program: Patient TB

He had an intracerebral hemorrhage from a right middle cerebral artery aneurysm four years previously. The aneurysm was clipped and he underwent a craniotomy for evacuation of the hematoma. There was a resulting dense left hemiplegia, left hemianopsia and multi-sensory neglect.

Because of his severe limitations, he was admitted to a local long-term care institution. Staff and family had much difficulty coping with his behaviours and supposedly changed personality that had resulted from the stroke. Although his residual medical problems were extensively documented in his charts, caregivers did not seem to realize that many of the inappropriate behaviours were neuropsychological rather than strictly characterological. A neuropsychological assessment of the cognitive deficits was never requested because the patient's verbal communication skills were well-preserved and because right-hemisphere cognitive disorders are not as apparent to caregivers as language disorders following left-hemisphere lesions. Consequently, it was felt that the initial referral for behavioural management should be preceded by a neuropsychological evaluation.

He presented as a restless and excitable man. Although labile, his expression of affect was rather flat. He had marked difficulties in the estimation of time and did not know his age. Although remarkably articulate, his thinking style was rapid and he haphazardly jumped to unrelated topics. His voice was raspy and choppy and his speech had poor prosody. He steadily increased the volume of his speech as he spoke, showing poor modulation.

All tests of right hemispheric functions showed marked impairments of both perceptual and constructional abilities. Drawings were scattered and fragmented, there was loss of spatial relations and organization of elements, faulty orientation and addition of lines to try and make drawings correct. When writing to dictation, he consistently wrote to the right side. When copying designs he neglected most details from the left side and when given reading material he ignored the left. Figures 2 and 3 give samples of the patient's responses showing evidence of perceptual neglect.

His impaired memory for location and for visual information seemed to be associated with his perceptual difficulties.

Testing revealed that Mr. L.S. performed normally on most tests of verbal functions. On tests of verbal memory, he was able to register, retain and recall material presented to him verbally.

ONCE THERE **LIVED A KING AND QUEEN IN**
A LARGE PALACE. **BUT THE KING AND QUEEN**
WERE NOT HAPPY. **THERE WERE NO LITTLE**
CHILDREN IN THE **HOUSE OR GARDEN.** ONE
DAY THEY FOUND **A POOR LITTLE BOY AND GIRL**
AT THEIR DOOR. **THEY TOOK THEM INTO THE**
BEAUTIFUL **PALACE AND MADE THEM THEIR**
OWN. THE **KING AND QUEEN WERE THEN**
HAPPY.

FIGURE 2: L.S. was asked to read the following story out loud. His
response is recorded as the darker typeset. He commented,
"Just doesn't make sense doctor...or is it me?"

Tests results, therefore, revealed severe cognitive deficits
consistent with brain damage lateralized to the right cerebral
hemisphere. The most impaired functions were: poor modulation of
affect; left unilateral multi-sensory neglect; perceptual and
constructional deficits. As a consequence of these deficits, his
memory for non-verbal tasks was greatly affected.

Because he did so well in verbal activities, the caregivers over-
estimated his abilities. His adjustment problems on the unit were
felt to be a consequence of a poor understanding by staff of the
effect that dramatic underlying perceptual deficits have on
psychosocial outcomes and every day behaviours.

Behavioural Management Program

In order to obtain a quantitative sample of aggressive behaviours, Mr.
L.S. was placed on a controlled behavioural management program. Staff
were given ABC charts and asked to record events that preceded the
aggressive behaviour, to give a description of the behaviour in as much
detail as possible and to document how they responded to the behaviour. A
sample of the first week baseline is illustrated in Table 2.

Over this period, 12 aggressive outbursts occurred. When reviewing
the charting it was apparent that many of the aggressive outbursts were
directly related to an underlying perceptual disorder of hemi-inattention.
A good example of this occurred when he was being returned to his room.
He became agitated and insisted he was on the wrong floor. After noting
the extent of his cognitive deficits in the neuropsychological assessment,

STIMULUS PRESENTED   PATIENT'S RESPONSE

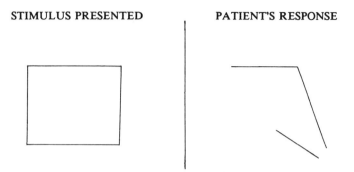

FIGURE 3: Example of Neglect. When asked to describe the stimulus
presented L.S. responded: "A bracket".

a likely explanation is that Mr. L.S. was neglecting the left side of the
halls as he was taken down to therapy. When he returned to his room he
was neglecting the opposite side of the halls and, in fact, perceiving a
completely different world. His poor memory for visual material may have
significantly compounded the problem. Perceptual deficits also played an
important role in other instances. Twice, the patient collided his
wheelchair with other residents. Here again it becomes obvious that his
perceptual deficit was the underlying trigger to an aggressive outburts.
The physical layout of his room was such that when he was put to bed, his
right side was facing the wall, thus making him vulnerable to apprehensive
reactions when staff entered his room (to give him medication as in
example 1) or when asking for his bell when it was attached to the left
bed rail (example 4).

The major focus of the behavioural treatment program for Mr. L.S. was
to educate family and staff about the nature of the cognitive deficits.
When given detailed feedback of the spared and impaired neuropsychological
functions, the caregivers readjusted their demands and expectations and
were quick to suggest creative solutions to bypass the left
hemi-inattentional problem. For example, important environmental changes,
especially in his room, were made to help him compensate for his
visuoperceptual problem. Following the intensive educational sessions and
the environmental adjustments, the aggressive outbursts subsided
significantly to about two outbursts the next week.

Once aggressive outbursts were less of a problem, a more standard
program of cognitive rehabilitation was initiated. Caregivers were taught

TABLE 2: BASELINE OBSERVATION PERIOD

<u>Date</u>	<u>Time</u>	Antecedent Behaviour	Problem Behaviour	Consequential Behaviour
06-05	0615	Staff entered room to give medication	"Are you against me too?... I want to get up.	Told nurse assigned to him would get him up. L.S. answered "No! not that big thing." referring to nurse B. Patient threw pillows on the floor.
	0830	Co-resident passed by L.S. in hallway and wheelchairs collided.	L.S. shouted to other resident - "get out of here...I'll punch you in the face!"	L.S. taken to his room. Upset by banging into furniture for 5 mins. Served breakfast. Co-operative and pleasant.
07-05	1300	L.S. returned to his room after session of physiotherapy on another floor.	L.S. shouted: "Take me to my floor this is not my floor!"	Nurse explained that this was his floor but L.S. insisted that this was not his floor.
	1600	L.S. in bed and shouting for nurse.	Shouting: "Where is my bell. I need my bell."	Nurse explained that call bell was attached to his bed rail. L.S. was told to stop disturbing other patients.
08-15	1015	Banged his wheelchair into another resident's wheelchair.	Screamed at other resident for being "stupid."	Nurse intervened and removed patient to room. Time spent with L.S. trying to answer his multiple questions.

to use frequent and consistent verbal cueing when communicating with him especially when helping him scan his environment systematically. Strategies to compensate for the hemi-inattention were developed. When reading, for example, the patient was given a visual cue to begin each line at the extreme left side of a page before proceeding and this improved his performance. This technique is referred to as anchoring. Even when anchoring is used, there is still a strong tendency for rapid drifting toward targets on the right side of the page. There is always a pull to the ipsilesional side of the brain damage. Patients with neglect can slow down their performance to a more even pace simply by saying the targets out loud. This has the effect of harnessing the speed of performance. This technique is called pacing. Three weeks after the management program was started, the behavioural outbursts were totally eliminated.

Discussion

Mr. L.S. had poor insight and could not describe his deficits to the caregivers. Having severe perceptual neglect, he was "unaware" of his deficits thus preventing insight into his condition. Patients with neglect typically resist awareness of their problems and, unfortunately, this is often seen as characterological resistance. A dramatic example of the neuropsychological basis for this lack of awareness is well illustrated in Figure 2. After neglecting the left half of a reading text, Mr. L.S. spontaneously added the comment: "Just doesn't make sense doctor...or is it me?" It is easy to understand how Mr. L.S. was constantly getting uninformed feedback for his inappropriate responses by caregivers who were equally unaware of how his severe perceptual disorder affected his everyday behaviours. It is no wonder that patients with hemi-inattention are said to be typically negativistic, stubborn and too often "act-out". In this case, the aggressive outbursts were eliminated, not so much because of direct training and therapy with him, but rather because of the readjustment and dramatic shift in the approach of the caregivers to the problem behaviours.

CONCLUSIONS

Prior to 1983, there had been no published studies on training family members to use behaviour management techniques with the impaired elderly (Haley, 1983). In contrast, the literature dealing with management of problem behaviours in children has been impressive over the last 25 years. Patterson (1987) believes that this is due to the attitude that behaviour problems in the elderly are chronic and untreatable. Too many caregivers still regard depression, incontinence, complaining, confusion and disorientation as appropriate behaviour for the elderly. Yet, such behaviours are not normal at any age. The reason that treatment of behavioural problems in the elderly is not provided in many cases is because caregivers know very little about the organic and environmental factors that trigger such behaviours (Hussian and Davis, 1985). The ultimate tragedy occurs when an elderly person is sent to an institution not because of health problems necessitating nursing care but because of a behavioural problem that could have been managed by the family, had they been properly informed and trained (Patterson, 1987).

Despite the exceptional growth of knowledge in cognitive psychology and clinical neuropsychology in the last decade, almost no attention has been given to treatment and management issues. There is still an excessive focus on diagnosis and description. In this chapter, I have tried to show that inappropriate behaviour in the cognitively-impaired elderly should be seen in the same way as inappropriate behaviour exhibited in other populations. Careful attention to context and to less readily observed variables such as cognitive dysfunctions is essential in understanding, predicting and controlling behaviours that negatively affect the patient's quality of life as well as that of the primary caregiver. Another important issue that was highlighted is that demented patients, once their medical status stabilizes, do much better in highly structured and predictable environments. This facilitates rote learning and cognitive "habilitation". When tasks are routine, structured and graded into small steps improvement in cognitive abilities is accelerated. Behavioural management is only successful in predictable environments where treatment is consistent and where as few caregivers as possible are involved. Such structure and consistency is almost impossible to achieve in large institutions where rotating staff is standard procedure. Behavioural management of cognitive disorders would be much more successful in smaller settings (eg. at home), where fewer caregivers are involved, provided that they receive appropriate home care, nursing care and respite services. The referral of cognitively-impaired elderly for management of disruptive behaviours is a reactive measure of desperation in many cases. The integration of cognitive sciences and behavioural management techniques would provide a more proactive approach to treatment and institutionalization might be postponed or even prevented.

No understanding of geriatric behaviour is complete without considering how cognitive disorders interact with the environment to produce behaviours that a caretaker can observe. Integration of principles from both the behavioural and neuropsychological domain holds great promise for improved management of disruptive behaviour in the cognitively impaired elderly.

ACKNOWLEDGEMENTS

Special thanks to Dr. Edith Kaplan, Dr. Morris Moscovitch and Dr. Mario Liotti for their helpful comments on this chapter.

REFERENCES

Broughton, R. (1975). Biorhythmic variations in consciousness and psychological functions. Canadian Psychological Review, 16, 217-239.

Hachinski, V.C., Lassen, N.A., Marshall, J. (1974). Multi-infarct dementia. A cause of mental deterioration in the elderly. Lancet, 2, 207-210.

Haley, W.E. (1983). A family-behavioural approach to the treatment of the cognitively impaired elderly. Gerontologist, 23, 18-20.

Hussian, R.A., Davis, R.L. (1985). Responsive Care: Behavioural Intervention with Elderly Persons. Champaign, Illinois: Research Press.

Jackson, G.M., Patterson, R.L. (1982). Behavioural principles and techniques. In Patterson, R.L., Dupree, L.W., Eberly, D.A., Jackson, G.M., O'Sullivan, M.J., Penner, L.A., Dee Kelly, C. (eds.). Overcoming Deficits Of Aging: A Behavioural Approach. New York: Plenum Press.

Kaplan, E. (1987). A Process Approach to Neuropsychological Assessment. Master Lecture, Annual Meeting of the American Psychological Association.

Le Bray, P.R. (1979). Geropsychology in long-term care settings. Professional Psychology, 70, 475-484.

Lezak, M.D. (1988). Brain damage is a family affair. Journal of Clinical and Experimental Neuropsychology, Vol. 10, No. 1, 111-123.

Miles, L., Dement, W. (1985). Sleep and aging. Sleep, 3, 119-220

Patterson, R. (1987). Family management of the elderly. In Carstensen, L.L., Edelstein, B.A. (eds.). Handbook Of Clinical Gerontology. New York: Pergamon Press.

Prigatano, G.P. (1986). Neuropsychological Rehabilitation After Brain
Injury. Baltimore: Johns Hopkins University Press.

Prinz, P., Raskind, M. (1978). Aging and sleep disorders. In Williams,
R., Karacan, I. (eds.). Sleep Disorders: Diagnosis And Treatment.
New York: Wiley, 303-321.

Wilson, B. (1987). Single-case experimental designs in
neuropsychological rehabilitation. Journal of Clinical and
Experimental Neuropsychology, Vol. 9, No. 5, 527-544.

Wilson, B. (1987). Rehabilitation of Memory. New York: Guilford Press.

CHAPTER 8

ISSUES OF CARE IN LONG-TERM SETTINGS

Sheldon S. Tobin, Ph.D.
Ringel Institute of Gerontology
School of Social Welfare
State University of New York
Albany, New York

Edelson and Lyons (1985), in the introduction to their excellent book Institutional Care of the Mentally Impaired Elderly, describe basic principles of working in institutional settings. They begin by admonishing readers not to confuse mental disease with "excess disability" that can be treated, particularly visual and auditory deficits. Care, they state must be "rehabilitative whenever possible, prosthetic whenever necessary, and at all times humane, identity-preserving, and ego-supporting" (p.XIX). They suggest that institutional arrangements "that support direct care staff (ie nursing staff) in establishing a supportive relationship with impaired residents focuses attention on how inter-disciplinary teams work" (p. XXI). Indeed, their message here is that the main purpose of teams, and mental health practitioners is to help in the structuring of ongoing supportive relationships between nursing staff and individual residents. The usefulness of sophisticated practitioners they say, is less in their one-to-one interaction with residents than in their educating and structuring of interaction between staff and residents.

Finally, they state: "As changes are made to meet the needs of the mentally impaired elderly, there will be resistance to change" (p. XXII) with the obvious challenge to professionals to facilitate change. Institutions must be assisted in changing so that they become settings where the identities of the residents do not have to change. Fortunately, mental health professionals are precisely those individuals who understand how hard it is to deal with resistance to change while at the same time knowing how to reduce that resistance.

One starting point in promoting institutional change is to educate nursing staff to consider the meaning of behaviour. What appears bizarre and aimless can become intelligible by understanding the motives and past coping style of the mentally impaired residents. Staff must come to understand what it means to live in a total institution (Goffman, 1961), a foreign environment where all residents are regulated by rules and procedures that govern daily activities. In an institution individuality may be lost, one's identity becoming attached to being one of the many disabled elderly people who need care. The aim of this chapter is to describe the impact of becoming institutionalized when old, factors which impede adaptation to institutionalized life, and issues of providing care.

BECOMING INSTITUTIONALIZED WHEN OLD

Although only about five percent of those sixty five and over reside in nursing homes, the probability of becoming institutionalized is high. In 1973 when four percent of the elderly were living in nursing homes, Kastenbaum and Candy (1973) referred to the "four percent fallacy" estimating the *probability* of institutionalization as twenty five percent; that is, for anyone surviving beyond sixty five there was a one in four chance of becoming institutionalized. Vencente, Wiley and Carrington (1979) estimated the probability at one in three. Moreover, the probability increases with age. Whereas, approximately two percent of those between sixty-five and seventy-four reside in long-term care facilities, the percentage is closer to twenty for those above eighty. Congruent with these increasing percentages with age, the average age of those in institutions is about eighty-five. It is of additional note that three of four nursing home residents have mental impairments (Larsen, Lo and Williams, 1986).

Tobin and Lieberman (1976) have examined the implications of institutionalization. In their study, reported in the book Last Home for the Aged: Critical Implications of Institutionalization, elderly individuals were followed from prior to admission through entering and living in long-term care facilities. At each point in time, these respondents, as well as respondents in community and institutional comparison samples, were extensively interviewed.

The study group consisted of eighty-five elderly individuals who were on waiting lists for entry into sectarian homes for the aged. Their average age was 79. They were interviewed four months before admission, two months after admission and again one year after admission. There were two comparison groups. The first consisted of thirty-seven elderly who had resided in the institutions for more than one year and the second was a community sample of forty. The community sample served as a baseline for studying the *process* of becoming waiting-list respondents.

The study employed a longitudinal design. Previous studies, have used a cross-sectional design to compare community and institutional samples (mostly of elderly in sectarian facilities, as discussed by Tobin and Lieberman, 1976). The investigators purposely selected sectarian homes for this study because they were judged to be the best of contemporary long-term care facilities, and hence best suited to evaluating the irreducible effects of institutional life. Differences in the two samples were attributed to living in the institution, although other factors may have been of even greater importance. These include population differences, preadmission factors and relocation effects.

Preadmission Factors

The investigators wanted to assess the fears which elderly individuals have of becoming institutionalized. For this purpose they used Kuypers' (1969) interview guide which taps into latent, as well as manifest, attitudes. Respondents voiced little manifest concern regarding their personal future and gave a positive appraisal of the sectarian institutions to which they would apply if that became necessary. Sample responses included feelings that old age homes were necessary, that the staff met the needs of residents, that a resident could maintain self-respect, and that the home provided companionship. To them, people who went into homes were different from themselves, but if they themselves were no longer independent "the home would be a necessary alternative." Contrasting results were obtained when latent attitudes were examined using a more focused interview. One respondent said "it would be giving up everything" and that she would go "only if helpless". Another compared it to "a jail," and a third to "a place to die." However, while it meant giving up everything, each indicated that they would enter the home, as had others before them, to assure survival. Given the latent attitudes of elderly toward these institutions before admission was even contemplated, it is not at all surprising that, if admission is later sought, the process is associated with negative psychological effects.

The investigators compared the three study groups on the four dimensions assumed to be most affected by actually living in an institutional environment, - cognition, emotional responsiveness, affect states and changes in the self-system. The waiting list group, compared to the community group, was more cognitively impaired, less emotionally responsive, had worsened affect states and negative changes in their self-esteem. Surprisingly, when compared to elderly who had lived in institutions, waiting list respondents had essentially the same psychological portraits. Cross-sectional comparison of the community, waiting list, and institutional samples corroborated this finding. (Lieberman, Prock, and Tobin, 1968). The waiting list and institutional samples were remarkably alike, and the community sample decidedly better, on all four psychological dimensions. If anything, the status of the institutional sample was better than that of the waiting list.

Differences between the demographically matched community and waiting list samples were attributable to the presence of adverse interpersonal changes in the previous three years. In particular, deteriorated inter-personal relationships, either had led to seeking institutional care or had followed the decision to seek care. This explanation contrasts with that of earlier cross-sectional studies which attributed such personality profiles to the effect of living in an institution.

The investigators were able to corroborate the importance of the role of interpersonal change when the latent meaning of applying to an institution was explored, using the reconstruction of the respondent's earliest memory as a projective test (see Tobin, 1972; Tobin & Etigson, 1968). Waiting list respondents expressed focal concerns of abandonment, separation from significant others without an expectation of reunion, feeling rejected and awaiting an uncertain fate. As Pincus (1968) points out however, this fear of abandonment is attenuated (or, if you will, defended against) by the verbalized manifest anticipation of physical care, security, and activities.

The Effects of Institutional Life

If, before admission, one experiences feelings of abandonment with an associated psychological portrait not unlike those who have resided in institutions, what changes can one expect to find when following the same people from preadmission to residence in the homes?

Using a longitudinal design, effects preceding admission and population differences could be controlled, (although relocation effects cannot be so readily dismissed). By following the same individuals from an average of four months before admission to two months after admission to the best of contemporary long-term care facilities, it was possible to come closer to answering: What are the irreducible effects of entering and living in long-term care institutions?

By two months after admission the typical institutional resident has been through what Jerome Grunes has called the First Month Syndrome, the transient, but severe, behavioural changes usually evidenced during the initial period after admission. Data gathered both before and after admission, suggested more stability than change by two months postadmission. Constrictions in cognition and affective responsiveness, evident prior to admission, persisted. There was a continuation (or stability) of moderate preadmission levels of well-being, anxiety and depression. Changes were limited to findings of increased hopelessness, increased bodily preoccupation, perceived reduced capacity for self-care and a lessening of affiliation in interaction with others. In contrast to the deselfing process which Goffman (1961) has described as occurring when entering a state mental hospital, the self-system remained remarkably intact and stable. Rosner (1968), using the interpersonal self-sort task, (the pool of forty eight self-descriptive items) confirmed the consistency in the self-view of the preadmission and post admission groups. In his study the only shift that did occur was on the affiliative-hostile dimension, indicating a perception of less friendliness and more hostility toward others.

Residents and their Families

Does the diminution in affiliation toward others suggest a decline in interaction with others? Data (from the Personal Resources Questionnaire) suggests that residents interact with a range of peers and staff, and also with family -- at least in the particular homes studied. With specific regard to the family, there is an amelioration of abandonment feelings (see, also, Smith and Bengtson, 1979), and a tendency toward mythicizing of living children. Although a child may still be alive and a frequent visitor, the increased psychological distance created by institution-alization and the need to preserve the self in the face of institutional demands and distance, may cause an exaggeration in the adaptive process of mythicizing a child. The exaggerated response is probably reinforced by the institutional environment where the coin of the realm is famous offspring who are attentive and caring and where family attention elevates personal prestige and encourages more attentive staff caring.

The Latent Meaning

To summarize the major findings of the Tobin and Lieberman study: entering and living in the institutional environment was not associated with changes that would support belief in the "destructiveness of institutions." However, the institution apparently "forces the adoption of the patient role, including increasing the preoccupation with bodily concerns and personal vulnerability, which, in turn, reduces the elderly resident's expectations for future gratifying experiences that can give purpose to life" (Tobin and Lieberman, 1976, p. 132).

The shift at the more latent level was not as modest as the manifest changes in psychological status. The individual's earliest memories revealed a significant shift toward the introduction of themes of mutilation and death. This shift in recollection sometimes occurred when the same incident was reported at two different times.

For example, before admission one elderly woman offered the following earliest memory: "I remember my mother. She had hair like braids, open and falling upon her shoulder. She was sitting up in her bed and near her on her table was a bottle of honey and I remember asking her for honey. That's all I remember-- nothing before and nothing behind. I still can see her sitting in bed. I must have been two years, two or three. Closer to two, I guess. But that's a picture I have."

After admission she recalled: "I remember my mother's death. I remember at least one moment of it. She had honey on her bed and I wanted some of that honey. I didn't really understand that she was dying. I was almost 3 years old. That's all I remember. I can see her face clearly even now. She had two braids hanging down. This picture is all I remember of her."

The contrast between the two memories suggests that a breakthrough of repression had occurred in which previously withheld, archaic material was now being expressed. It would appear that in the first report the pain of mother's death was defended against, a pain which broke through in the second telling of the same incident.

More often, the loss associated with institutionalization was associated with a shift in the content of early memory. For example, one respondent, while on the waiting list, recounted this earliest memory:

"I liked to go swimming and mother wouldn't let me. Once I stood on the pier and fell in. I remember how they took me out and took me to my mother. That's all I remember. I wasn't sick."

But after admission he reported:

"Didn't have coffins in the old country like they do here. My father died. I remember my sister was still a breast baby...It was a cold day. My mother said don't go. But he was a stubborn man and so he got pneumonia and died."

Contrasts with thematic changes in the control groups suggest that one-third would not have shifted to these themes of more narcissistic loss had they not entered the homes. The shift may be understood as specifically related to entering and living in a total institutional environment with sick elderly in a home that is to be the last one. With such a significant shift, from abandonment to increased vulnerability, it was indeed surprising that so little change was observed in manifest psychological status. Most likely, the ability to successfully contain, to defend against, the latent meanings is a function of the excellent care found in the best of contemporary long-term care facilities. Yet even these facilities exact their toll, as reflected in the latent meaning of institutional life itself, in the adoption of the patient role, a lessening of futurity, and portraying oneself as less affiliative in relation to others.

At the End of One Year

By the end of one year postadmission, approximately one-half of the the sample had either died (fifteen percent) or had sharply deteriorated (thirty-three percent). Those we were able to interview again showed only a lessening of affiliation in relation to others and a lessening of body preoccupation. All other measures showed no change. This pattern of stability, with only focal changes in affiliation and body preoccupation, among the intact survivors, masks the above-noted global outcomes; forty-one of the eighty-five had died or had become extremely deteriorated. It is impossible to know to what extent these forty-one would have shown these outcomes had they not entered the homes. Although similar outcomes were found for eighteen percent of the community sample, such outcomes were found for forty seven percent of the institutional control sample. The latter statistic suggests no excess morbidity and mortality for those who entered the homes.

Predicting Vulnerability to the Stress of Institutionalization

The intact and non-intact respondents did not differ in age, but they did differ in living arrangements prior to admission. Of the eighty five respondents, seventeen lived in nursing homes prior to admission. The other sixty five lived with others or alone in non-institutional settings. Of those admitted from nursing homes, seventy-seven percent were in the non-intact group. Relocation from a nursing home to a home for the aged is obviously associated with more negative outcome than relocation into the home from independent community living. Yet those admitted from nursing homes were similar to those admitted from the community on most of our measures. For example, they differed neither on functional adequacy nor in the severity or number of events leading to the decision to seek institutional care. However, it is also possible that their deterioration partially resulted from the earlier relocation. They had to adapt to the stress of two relocations in a rather brief time interval. This double relocation may explain the few differences that were found between those elderly admitted from the community and those from the nursing homes who tended to be more passive, to use more denial, and to have a lowered sense of futurity, characteristics that, in many ways, reflect an institutional profile. Their lower anxiety level and greater comfort in relating to the interviewer may have related to their

assurance of care while in the nursing home and to being further along in
their resolution of the issues of loss and abandonment, than the
respondents who were admitted directly from the community.

When the groups were compared on nine predictors of outcome to stress
(i.e. functional capacities, affects, hope, the self-system, personality
traits, reminiscence, coping with the impending event, interpersonal
relations and accumulated stress), only one dimension, the personality
trait of passivity was a specific predictor of vulnerability to the stress
of institutionalization. In other words, passivity was predictive of
increased morbidity and mortality for those in stable environments (also
see Turner, Tobin & Lieberman, 1972).

When residents on the waiting list were assessed for how they were
mastering the impending event of institutionalization, it was found that
those who transformed the situation so as to make the move totally
voluntary, and also perceived the relocation environment as ideal, were
those most likely to survive intact through one year following admission.
This kind of magical story, as well as aggressiveness and hopefulness (but
not the absence of clinical depression) were found to enhance adaptation
in three additional relocation situations which are described in the book
by Lieberman and Tobin (1982), The Experiences of Old Age.

A CARING ENVIRONMENT

Not unexpectedly, the quality of the psychosocial environment is a
predictor of outcome. Nursing homes, that individualized care, contained
warm staff-resident relationships and enhanced autonomy were associated
with more intact survivorship. This was most clear in the fourth study
reported in The Experiences of Old Age, the *en masse* relocation of
four-hundred and twenty-seven state mental hospital patients to one
hundred and forty-two nursing and boarding homes. The relocated group had
a death rate, one year after relocation, of eighteen percent, and the
carefully matched control group of one hundred, who were not relocated,
had a death rate, in the same interval, of only five percent. Those who
died following the relocation were likely to have entered facilities of
poor psychosocial quality. While all relocations are associated with
adverse reactions to stress, excess mortality among these relocated state
mental hospital patients was largely a result of their initial debilitated
physical status. Reactions to relocation of less debilitated elderly
persons, such as those in our study of institutionalization in sectarian
homes, are likely to be less extreme. Rather than death, excess morbidity
was prominent among those with the worst outcomes.

The obvious conclusion to be drawn from studies of the impact of psychosocial environment on outcome, is that any and all enhancements of quality will facilitate adaptation. Indeed, the psychosocial quality of environments is the strongest predictor of relocation outcome. Simply put, the poorer the quality, the worse the outcome. The next strongest predictor relates to individual characteristics, specifically an ability to magically master the situation. Kahana, Liang and Felton (1980) found that morale level after admission correlated better with individual characteristics of need for affect expression (akin to aggressiveness) and institutional control (akin to magical mastery) than it did with congruence, or "person-environment fit," (although person-environment fit made a modest difference). Those who wished to be separate from others had better morale when they went to a nursing home that permitted greater separation. Still, the most significant predictor of adverse reactions to relocation, is an inadequate relocation environment.

Pre-Admission Preparation

Whose responsibility is it to mobilize aggressiveness, enhance magical coping and instill hopefulness before admission? When admission occurs quickly, as when the resident arrives directly from the hospital, it is not possible for the staff of the facility to work directly with the resident before admission. If there is any waiting period before admission, staff must prepare residents-to-be for the move.

Dealing with the First Month Syndrome

After admission, the first month syndrome of disorientation, depression and other symptoms of extreme distress can be expected. It is essential that the staff assume that this is a temporary state which generally will diminish as the resident adapts to the new environment. Only if this assumption is made will new residents be helped to recover from the initial shock of social dislocation. Indeed, the quality of an institution can be determined by the level of the staff's awareness and acknowledgement of the initial first month syndrome. Facilities in which staff say "everybody does fine when they first come in," are likely to be precisely those which are associated with greater deterioration following the relocation.

There are many ways to assist the transition. For example, one facility, with which the author was associated for many years, a treatment, or more accurately a service plan, was developed at admission, in which the staff attempted to anticipate the course of adjustment and to minimize distress. This approach often led to creative solutions to difficult problems. For example, whenever a resident could be placed with

a roommate who needed to nurture a more dependent partner the marriage
was made. Every attempt was made to integrate these residents, and avoid
segregation, despite difficulties.

Acknowledging Irreversible Effects

As discussed previously, even in the best of facilities, there are
irreversible effects of becoming a resident in a total institution.
Whereas, at a latent level, the inner experience will be that of being
more physically vulnerable and closer to death, these feelings can be
contained. Most residents of facilities of high psychosocial quality are
able to preserve their identity, their sense of self-sameness, albeit with
less hopefulness, with less of an expectation that they can make a
fulfilling future for themselves, and with a greater preoccupation with
bodily concerns. Unavoidable, even with only a modicum of cognitive
intactness, is the awareness that to live in a long-term-care facility is
to live with other old, impaired persons with whom you are grouped
together in daily routines. Only through individualizing care can these
feelings be counteracted. And it is through the hands-on staff that
individualizing of care can occur.

Working with Staff

Echoing Edelson and Lyons, an institutional orientation to enhancing
residents' functioning must penetrate interactions between residents and
staff at all levels. Such penetrations occur through staff's understanding
of resident's behaviour, but there are many barriers that must be overcome
if there are to be accurate appraisals of behaviours, particularly of
demented residents. Staff, like family, find it difficult to understand
how seemingly pathological processes are actually functional. Aggressiveness, nastiness and even paranoid behaviours are often facilitatory of
adaptation to stress. In this regard, Brody and her associates (Brody,
Kleban, Lawton and Silverman, 1971; Kleban, Brody and Lawton, 1971) found
that excess disabilities in activities of daily living could only be
decreased among those residents who were more assertive.

Staff must learn to understand, tolerate and even nurture verbally
abusive, aggressive and paranoid behaviours directed at them by
residents. Obviously this is a difficult task, a task too difficult for
some staff. It is also a task that is not assumed by staff in many
facilities, where even the most minor of deviations from ideal compliance
and gratefulness are not tolerated. An illustration of intolerance of
the non-ideal resident was provided by a graduate social work student. For
an assignment in a course on psychopathology, he chose to write-up the
case of a sixty-seven year old woman who was a resident in a nursing
home. The student, a minister in his fifties whose newly self-appointed

ministry was to work with and for the elderly, prepared an excellent case report.

> Mrs. G. was always self-centered and impulsive. She had, for example, abandoned two children, one with each of two husbands that she left. A third husband had died within the previous two years and she had had a stroke. The student voiced his concern that Mrs. G. was labelled as "a histrionic who is always manipulating and demanding." He was concerned that staff members were vilifying this lady who needed care and attention for her recovery. When I asked the student to repeat his description of Mrs. G. he became flustered and responded that she is self-centered, but then added that "that is no reason to treat her so badly." "So," I asked "is the judgement of the staff wrong?" He was unwilling at this time, to accept that there was agreement in the diagnosis and continued to focus on her bad treatment. After returning to Mrs. G. in the next three class sessions, it became apparent to the student that the diagnosis was correct and that Mrs. G. was neither an admirable lady nor particularly likeable. Moreover, he began to realize that the task of the facility and the staff, and especially his task, because he was now Mrs. G.'s caseworker, was to help her to be who she is. It was not love she needed, and indeed he could not love her despite his Christian beliefs, but help to retain her persistent self-centered identity. His supervisor realized the task and began to understand how her own dislike for Mrs. G. caused her to ally herself with the other vituperative staff members. Fortunately, she was then able to reestablish a professional perspective and to assist the student, as well as staff, to accept Mrs. G. for the person she is. A few weeks later, the student thanked me, and said that Mrs. G. was making a splendid recovery but is no more likeable.

The supervisor, the student and some staff were sufficiently professional and mature to accept Mrs. G.'s distasteful behaviour. It would have been more difficult if Mrs. G. had been verbally abusive, rather than self-aggrandizing and demanding of attention. Similarly, staff must learn that magical thinking of residents can also be functional for adaptation and survival. Beliefs in magical mastery must be encouraged, at least until the point of imminent and extreme danger. Goldfarb (1959), a psychoanalyst with over thirty years as a psychiatric consultant in a nursing home, based his psychotherapy with the institutional elderly on "overinflating beliefs in environmental mastery."

Yet, lower level staff cannot begin to understand the meanings of these seemingly pathological behaviours unless professionals do. Professionals, however, can too easily interpret facilitatory mechanisms as psychopathological if they use models developed for younger persons.

Professionals are often taught that good coping necessitates realistic appraisals of one's capacities, and that abusive behaviour towards others reflects bad object relations. Although such generalizations may generally be correct, they may be completely wrong when applied to the very old, particularly when they are under duress.

As Edelson and Lyons (1985), and Lyons (1982) point out, staff must learn that bizarre behaviours often have meanings related to the striving for preservation of self. Once this principle is understood, it becomes increasingly possible to see continuity between bizarre behaviour and pre-morbid personality traits. In turn, as the bizarre behaviours become intelligible, the staff can tolerate, and when appropriate encourage, seemingly aberrant behaviours that help the patient be him or herself.

It is not easy for staff to be objective. They have good reasons for feeling angry, helpless and demoralized, frustrated and even betrayed (Dobrof 1983). Feelings of anger towards residents is reflected in comments such as "How can he say these things to me, after all I have done for him?" Anger toward the family may be justified in a comment such as, "Don't they even care about that old man? He probably just sits there like that because they never visit him." Thoughts about the other staff members and supervisors include, "They leave all the dirty work for me; nobody ever shows any appreciation around here." Feelings of helplessness and demoralization are reflected in, "It doesn't seem to matter what we do, they never get any better." Should not the aide feel frustrated when saying to herself, "I must have explained that to her six times already"? The terrible feeling of betrayal is captured by the comment, "After everything I have done for her, she doesn't even know who I am." There is obviously no easy way to reduce these painful feelings, however, it is necessary to provide to the hands-on staff a sense of efficacy and potency.

Burnside (1981), divided these techniques for managing patients with cognitive impairments into three categories: techniques for the helper, techniques for memory development and techniques for manipulation of the environment. Her "bedside" helper recommendations include: reinforce reality; use touch; support denial if it is therapeutic; approach slowly; do not argue; do not take the client's behaviour personally; do not try to alter long-standing personality patterns; use both short and frequent contacts; reduce the client's need to employ functions which have been lost; identify feelings and help clients to express them; assess physical and psychological liabilities early; preserve functions; gain knowledge of premorbid personality characteristics; talk with the patient and not about her or him; gain the attention of the patient; use appropriate affection and praise; enhance self-expression; do not push and give orders; become aware of your tone of voice and approach and of how the client will respond and react; do not take problems home; and eliminate or reduce unexpected situations that cause duress.

Marchico-Greenfield (1986) advocated similar techniques for facilitating communication between impaired elderly residents and their families: be natural; share ideas, thoughts and problems; speak more slowly, more loudly, vividly, concretely, descriptively and clearly; choose topics that are interesting, familiar and important; avoid rapid topic changes; keep talking whenever appropriate; accept any form of communication; use and encourage gestures; give hints to facilitate the message; allow extra time for responding; accept answers which are a close approximation; elicit and prompt answers without forcing them; allow for warmup by not beginning visits with crucial messages; allow for turn-taking during the conversations if possible; do not over-correct; acknowledge breakdowns in communication; when all else fails, provide things to talk about; be sensitive to changes in attitude and energy; if misunderstood, revise and repeat what has been said; if unsure of what was said, seek clarification; summarize conversations frequently; if one approach is not working, try another; do not speak for the resident; include the resident in all discussion; give the resident choices and facilitate all decisions; promote reminiscing.

Reducing duress is particularly important. Situations that provoke agitation, including most new situations, must be recognized. Obviously, when the impaired resident cannot communicate the source of the agitation, disorganized and aberrant behaviour is likely to escalate. While one may ask whether staff become more comfortable, more competent and feel more efficacious in working with demented patients, staff education in communication is very helpful. It is possible to enhance the functioning and feelings of staff, especially through the support and reassurance of the more senior and/or prestigious professional staff. The more that staff are expected to put out, the more they must be nourished.

Burnside has suggested strategies to enhance memory development, including approaches which are appropriate for reality orientation groups, as well as for interaction outside of groups. For example, she suggests providing sufficient cues to aid memory and orientation (e.g. props to indicate change of season); consistent cues that encourage recognition instead of recall; avoiding pressure to perform; being sure to communicate what the resident is expected to remember; and being sure that familiar objects, reaffirming the continuity of the sense of self, are on display.

Environmental manipulations are rather obvious such as using a night light; bright colors and decoration; color coded doors; keeping the same staff working with individuals; providing a safe, non-threatening environment that is not too boring but not over stimulating; providing clocks and calendars; and making special efforts to provide a milieu that reduces sundowners syndrome.

Behavioural Interventions

In vogue now are behavioural interventions. What is meant by behavioural approaches to intervention? Simply stated, interaction between the resident and the environment is first analyzed for factors that encourage dysfunctional behaviour; then, new kinds of interactions are substituted that encourage restoration of ADL (activities of daily living) functioning; and, lastly, improvement in ADL is charted (Pinkston, Levitt, Green, Linsk and Rzepnicki 1982). However, behaviourists use different terminology: environmental contingencies that reinforce dysfunctional behaviour are analyzed; new contingencies introduced; and targeted behaviour is charted for extinction of dysfunctional aspects and for increased frequency of functional aspects. Regardless of language, successful restoration of functioning has been demonstrated for a diversity of deficits including, an inability to use eating utensils by use of one-to-one skill training at every meal; daytime urinary incontinence for wheelchair-bound residents, by use of a bell with toileting at fixed two-hour intervals; and incoherent speech, by constant positive reinforcement of intelligible speech, while ignoring unintelligible speech.

If the successes are so impressive, why have behavioural approaches not been embraced with enthusiasm? Too often, a graduate student in psychology has applied the intervention. Thus, he or she has devoted a great deal of time to an individual resident, while providing relief for overburdened staff who invariably are delighted to have the added, and optimistic, assistance. Unfortunately, when the student leaves, the intervention ceases. Also, the most successful interventions have occurred in facilities of the poorest quality where any intervention is likely to have a positive impact on function and behaviour. Giving residents a choice of two dinner entrees for example, can indeed be a potent force in a facility of poor quality! (Rodin and Langer, 1977). Even under the best of circumstances, in facilities of high quality and with excellent staff training as behavioural modifiers, improvements do not continue beyond the period of intervention. Unless sustained prosthetic environments are developed to reinforce desired behaviours, reestablished functioning will decay and previously extinguished behaviours will return (Lindsley, 1964).

Despite the exaggerated optimism regarding behavioural approaches, some important lessons have been learned. The presence of eager graduate students is immensely valuable for improving morale and performance on units of cognitively impaired residents. This was certainly so for example, on the unit where a doctoral student applied a behavioural approach to helping residents to empty their bladders on a fixed schedule. During the period that he was on the unit, morale was noticeably better. Staff liked the affable student who was always courteous and respectful and, also, was most willing to lend a hand when called upon, to help lift a resident or to carry a tray. In turn, only through their assistance, was he able to show that a bell that rang on a fixed schedule, followed by the staff assisting the resident to urinate successfully, kept residents dry. When he left, however, the staff felt an emptiness and soon reverted to letting residents become incontinent during the day. Only by assigning a staff member to attend to the resident's needs when the bell rang, would it have been possible to maintain this program.

Clearly, unless appropriate levels of reinforcement are maintained, both outside of the minutes or hours of a formal program, and beyond a fixed period of weeks or months, improvements disappear. But probably the most important lesson is that unless staff members are taught why what they are doing is particularly helpful to the resident, there is no generalization. When teaching staff help front-line personnel understand the reason for interventions, they provide both the prerequisite knowledge for their actions and the support, and necessary nourishment, for the arduous tasks of caring for cognitively impaired residents.

Because apparently aberrant behaviour may have an important self-sustaining function for an individual, its purpose should be sought before behavioural techniques are introduced to extinguish it.

A poignant example occurred in a home for the aged, when a graduate student wished, without knowledge of its underlying meaning, to change the fondling behaviour of Mrs. L., a rather confused female resident. Mrs. L.'s fondling of the breasts and genitalia of other women was particularly offensive to staff members. By the time the student arrived, however, the consulting psychiatrists had explained to staff members that Mrs. L.'s fondling was a reflection of her relationship with her deceased husband. Her daughter had related how her parents were such a loving couple that they always held hands and were constantly touching and gently petting each other. Mrs. L. was actually rather terrified of men and thus sought out women to replace her lost and needed tactile contact. The consultant's approach was to facilitate her behaviour in more adaptive form, encouraging her to form a tactile relationship with a narcissistic woman who appreciated Mrs. L.'s attention, and to confine the fondling, as much as possible, to private areas in the facility. In the consultant's view, had the fondling behaviour been extinguished by behavioural interventions, Mrs. L.'s deterioration would have likely rapidly accelerated.

In summary, behaviourist interventions must not be targeted on behaviours that preserve the self but, rather, on behaviours that diminish the self. For reinforcement to be effective, procedures must be incorporated into the service plan and be part of the everyday routine. Implementation must be by staff who, regardless of specific discipline, assure the creation of a prosthetic environment for each resident.

Group Interventions

In common with behavioural approaches, group interventions must also be augmented by a continuous prosthetic environment. For example, structural change of the physical environment can enhance and complement therapeutic programs. In one home, a wander-proof lounge was developed which allowed wandering residents to spend two hours a day roaming freely while participating in structured programming. The residents were thereby safely off their floors, providing a needed respite for floor staff (Malzer and Cox, 1987). Such a lounge becomes a stable environment in which wanderers can freely explore many artifacts of interest. Purposeful behaviour is encouraged, and participants urged to reminisce in groups, forming coherent images and expressions of the past. In this specific instance, when participants returned to their floor, the staff reported less random wandering and enhanced sleeping patterns.

THE FAMILY AND THE INSTITUTIONALIZED IMPAIRED ELDERLY

By the time a decision is made to institutionalize an elderly member, the family often feels conflicted - relieved, but guilty and inadequate. Moreover, they may experience rage at themselves for being inadequate and at the elderly person for inducing feelings of inadequacy. Too often workers focus only on the family's feelings of guilt, omitting the accompanying feelings of inadequacy, rage and sense of relief which occurs after institutionalization. One outcome of a narrowly focused view of the emotional conflicts in families is that staff may then seek to reassure family members of the wisdom of their action and give them subtle, or not so subtle, messages that it is not necessary to visit so much, thereby reducing the pain of visiting a relative who is quickly deteriorating and who may not even recognize them. Visits by family members, however, are particularly important because of the effects of becoming institutionalized when old.

When an elderly person is institutionalized in a long-term-care setting, the de-selfing process can be attenuated, in part, by interaction with family members. For example, a severely confused elderly person may seem to be totally unaware of the family visitor at the time of the visit. Shortly thereafter, however, they may become quite agitated, probably reflecting an awareness of, and reaction to, the visit.

Despite its importance to the resident, a visit can be quite upsetting to the family visitor and serve only to heighten his or her feelings of guilt, impotence and rage. Unless someone explains the specific meaningfulness and importance of the visit to the family they may reduce their visiting, further assaulting the emotional state of the elderly resident.

For those without family, or with families who are unable or unwilling to visit, the de-selfing process can accelerate. Not only are these residents without the benefit of significant others who can reinforce the self, but staff are less likely to see the resident as a real person. One remedy for this situation, developed by the author, is to use volunteers who commit themselves to consistent ongoing visits to the same resident. In the author's experience, by careful preparation and pairing, such visiting persists for a long time.

A Structured Approach to Families

In the best of institutions, family visiting is encouraged. Unfortunately, however, as the residential population inevitably deteriorates and becomes more mentally impaired, family visits to the resident tend to decrease. In the author's program, staff attempted to maintain visiting patterns by developing family groups, comprised of family members of new residents. While these groups did keep families involved in the home, relatives of more confused residents did not necessarily visit either the floor of their resident family member, or the resident, even though they were in the building (Safford, 1980). In withdrawing from interaction with deteriorating residents, some family members simply deny that their visiting has lessened, others become upset at their inability to tolerate the deterioration, while still others vociferously blame the home for causing the deterioration.

Ubiquitous among families is anger toward themselves and toward the resident that is frequently displaced onto the home and its staff. A successful approach to families must therefore allow for the expression of displaced rage, since this is more beneficial to family members than rage turned inward and certainly better than rage expressed toward the resident.

To operationalize such a philosophy, a home and its staff must be able to accept the anger of both residents and family members. Aggressiveness by residents, (often characterized by staff in such terms as "complaining" "griping" and "bitchiness") may then be more helpfully and accurately perceived as facilitating adaptation, and its absence a cause for alarm. Moreover, unless complaining is tolerated, and even encouraged, staff and administration may become complacent, promoting the dominance of administrative needs over resident needs.

From a more psychodynamic perspective, families develop unconscious relationships (transference) to the institution, which include both positive and negative projections (Gendel and Reiseer, 1981; Reider, 1953; Safirstein, 1967; Wilmer, 1962; Van Eck, 1972). In other words the home becomes both the symbolic and real life-sustaining, all-giving, all-loving other, while concurrently being perceived to be the life-impeding other that is the cause of the present and future deterioration of their family member. To direct this institutional transference more usefully, the author developed a structured approach to the institutional psychosocial environment. Simply put, a split transference was fostered, wherein a unit social worker became the all-giving, all-loving other, and administrative personnel the life-impeding others.

The hiring of the social workers was a careful process in which persons were sought who were genuinely altruistic and giving individuals. With the unit worker, family members discussed the concrete needs of the resident. When, for example, a cherished, forty-year old, thread-worn and torn sweater was missing, the social worker could assure a family member who was totally convinced that it was stolen or lost in the laundry, that every means would be taken to recover it. Often, of course, the confused resident had misplaced it or, at other times, the ancient garment had simply dissolved in the process of being cleaned and had been replaced by housekeeping with a sweater in better repair. After the worker's assurance, the family could leave the home knowing that the worker would devote herself, or himself, to searching for the missing cherished sweater. Their sense of personal inadequacy and guilt was thus partially alleviated through projection onto the worker, of feelings and actions of unconditional caring and love for the family member in the home.

The psychodynamics in the relationship between family member and worker are indeed complex. Initially, at the point of admission, the resident represses or suppresses feelings of abandonment and focuses on how the home will assure survival, and provide opportunities for activity and socializing with peers. Concurrently, family members initially recognize that "It's time..."; that is, that "It's time to live in a nursing home." By choosing a facility of excellent quality, guilt is assuaged and the family perceive the staff of the home, particularly intake social workers, as assuring that the correct decision for placement has been made and that the home will appropriately respond to their elderly family member's needs.

After admission, however, families begin to observe the vicissitudes of the first month syndrome. During this early, post-admission phase, the family's initial relief from the burden of caregiving is replaced by a growing awareness that the institution is more impersonal in its caring than they admitted when seeking admission. They further realize that their family member is but one of many sick and deteriorating elderly for whom the home provides care. Using the proposed model of intervention, the worker is inserted into this disillusioning process so that fantasies of the home's special concern and caring for "my husband", "my wife", "my mother", "my father", "my aunt", "my uncle", "my grandma" or "my grandpa" become re-established. At this stage, the family perceives the worker as different from all other workers in the home. They see her as taking a special interest in their family member. Most families rationalize that the special interest, concern and care of the worker is because "mama, after all, is a special person" although in reality mama may actually be only a shell of her former self and not very lucid. A concurrent rationalization is that "I am a special person because of all I have done for mama." Thus the worker is perceived as not unlike an ideal family member, an extension of self who is not only always at mother's bedside, but who loves mother as the family does. The attention and caring is fantasized as stemming from unconditional love and certainly not because it is paid employment. Thus, for some family members, the worker becomes the perfect child, creating in the real child a sense of satisfaction that mother's needs are being met with tender loving care.

With this approach, rage toward the home may subside somewhat, but it is not completely extinguished. The worker can assist in containing the rage through her or his own actions, and through explanations regarding how good the home truly is. Yet the displaced rage of the family never subsides completely because the source of the anger i.e. at oneself for abandoning mother, or at mother for evoking feelings of inadequacy, shame and guilt, never fully resolves. The rage is not generally directed toward the all-loving and all-caring worker but rather toward an authority figure, for example, the charge nurse, the chief of social service, or the administrators, who became the "bad" other who they perceive as causing all their woes. The covert feeling about these authority figures is that "if they only cared enough, they would make her well again." Such projections have often taken the form of irrational tirades, particularly when a symbiotic relationship exits between daughter and mother. But if the staff come to understand that the interaction between daughter and mother is helpful for the maintenance of the mother's sense of self-identity such verbal abuses of staff become tolerable. The staff can appreciate that the irrational abuse is an expression of the daughter's internal state, particularly her own fear of personal dissolution, when observing deterioration in her mother. Maintaining staff tolerance is not an easy task! As already emphasized, it can only be accomplished if staff are supported and nourished by administration so that they can withstand personal abuse.

Although a formal evaluation of this technique has not been undertaken, there was a consensus among all levels of staff that this type of structuring of services was a great improvement over previously used methods. The long tradition of centralized social services and activity programs, increasingly made less sense as the residential population deteriorated. As a result, more of the activity programs occurred on the floor. The worker, by virtue of her close working alliance with the families, incorporated them into the service plan and sometimes into assisting with caregiving.

A significant shift occurred over time, from a perception of staff and families that the social service department was part of administration and separate from the daily care of all residents, to a perception of the department as intimately related to even the most tedious of nursing procedures. When the worker assumed responsibility for explaining to a daughter why mother was not bathed immediately on wetting her undergarments and had to wait a short while for the aide who was then busy, all floor staff appreciated the assistance. Also appreciative were personnel in housekeeping and dietary services who formerly were approached by families primarily to be criticized. The worker's explanations of the duties and concerns of these personnel led to a better relationship with families, as well as between these personnel and administrative staff.

With the apparent success of the program, those administrative staff who were the targets of criticism, and sometimes vociferous, verbal abuse by families, were better able to tolerate these behaviours. Sharing of information among the workers and administrative staff led to a sense of partnership in which each set of personnel could perceive and understand their role in encouraging successful visiting and in humanizing care. Clearly, more families were involved with not only their resident family member but also more staff members of the home.

A FINAL COMMENT

Individualizing care for mentally impaired residents is indeed difficult. Yet it can be accomplished by understanding the motives and needs of each resident. Administrators and staff members must be receptive, or made receptive, to modifying practices and policies. Mental health professionals have an important role to perform in facilitating programs and individual care that will help each mentally impaired resident to preserve a sense of self.

The loss of self must be the primary focus. Cohen and Eisdorfer (1986) entitled their book on how to help families cope with a member who has Alzheimer's disease, The Loss of Self. Early in the book, they quote one victim: "Most people expect to die someday, but whoever expected to lose their self first." Lyons (1982), who cared at home for his wife who was a victim of the disease, observed her struggle to preserve her feelings of self, and described her thoughts in his own words. In a powerful statement, he gives us a poignant description of what it means to be a victim of Alzheimer's Disease. He highlights the importance of helping his wife to remain the same person, aiding her in doing the same things she has always done, and he demonstrates that seemingly bizarre and aimless activities are indeed often purposeful.

"For me, this is a life and death struggle from which I can collapse into crushing defeat and withdrawal, or I can be aroused to a fever pitch of agitation and frustration expressed in pacing, in tearing at my clothing, repetitive movements or sounds. You may think I am completely out of it, but if you watch me closely I may startle you with my awareness of, for example, the danger of walking down steps or the presence of a person, or I may be searching for a person or an activity which I usually do around this time of day. My attempts to indicate to you that I am missing something may not make sense, and you may write off my behaviour as the meaningless actions of a person who lacks memory and does not know what time it is, or where he is. Yet, inside, in my own perception of things, I am reaching for something very real, and trying in my own way to find it or to get you to help me.

You may fail to help me do what I can do, by not taking the time and trouble to discover this. It is much simpler to do things for me, because that way is quicker and surer and more efficient. But, do you realize that this may make me more confused, frustrated, sometimes resistive and resentful. Sure I am cognitively impaired, but that means you have to use your ingenuity and your patience to help me to clue into what you want me to do and to try to understand what I want to do.

Then I face the opposite kind of problem in which because of my inability, you may think I lack motivation and therefore you try to pull or push me into doing things in the belief that somehow, if I am not pushed into them and I am not engaged, you are colluding in making me more helpless.

But it is not only your misperceptions of me which add to my problems. It is also what you are feeling deep inside of you, because I know you are terrified by my losses. You are well-meaning, good-intentioned,

normally kind and considerate. But inside, you cannot help but feel
not just pity, but some revulsion; not just empathy but also some
rejection.

When I am incontinent, I do not like it. I can still experience shame
and embarrassment. But I am helpless to protect myself against it,
especially when you are not tuned to my signals when I want to go. I
am also helpless to protect myself against your annoyance and disgust.
Do you know how dependent I am upon you to protect my dignity which
is so often assaulted?

I know that you really cannot cut down all the barriers that isolate
me. But you can look for those things which reduce my frustration,
which help smooth the way in the face of what confounds me, if you
take the time and make the effort to help me bridge, at least
partially, that cognitive gap which separates me from reality. I am
not gone, I am here.

Do you really know how terribly alone I am, closed in and cut off from
so many people and so many things around me? How I try, and why I
cry? For God's sake, help me in my terrible isolation. That is my
cry and my pain at its most raw and elemental level" (pp. 3-6).

REFERENCES

Brody, E.M., Kleban, M.H., Lawton, M.P., Silverman, H.A. (1971). Excess
    disabilities of mentally impaired aged: impact of individualized
    treatment. Gerontologist, 11, 124-133.

Burnside, I.M. (1981). Nursing and the Aged. New York: McGraw-Hill.

Cohen, D., Eisdorfer, C. (1986). The Loss of Self. New York: Norton
    Publishing.

Dobrof, R. (1983). Training Workshops on Caring for the Mentally
    Impaired Elderly. New York: The Brookdale Center on Aging of Hunter
    College.

Edelson, J.S., Lyons, W. (1985). Institutional Care of the Mentally
    Impaired Elderly. New York: Van Nostrand Reinhold Company.

Gendel, M.H., Reiseer, D.E. (1981). Institutional Countertransference.
    Am. J. of Psychiaty, 138, 508-511.

Goffman, E. (1961). Asylums. Chicago: Adline Publishing Company.

Goldfarb, A.I. (1959). Minor maladjustment in the aged. In Arieti, S. (ed.). American Handbook of Psychiatry. New York: Basic Books.

Grunes, J.M. (1982). Reminiscence, regression and empathy - a psychotherapeutic approach to the impaired elderly. In Greenspan, S.I. and Pollock, G.H. (eds.). The Course of Life. Washington, D.C., National Institute of Mental Health, 545-548.

Kahana, E., Liang, J., Felton, B.J. (1980). Alternative models of person-environment fit: prediction of morale in three homes for the aged. J. Gerontol, 35, 584-595.

Kastenbaum, R., Candy, S. (1973). The four percent fallacy: a methodological and empirical critique of extended care facility population statistics. Int. J. Aging and Hum. Dev., 4, 15-21.

Kleban, M.H., Brody, E.M., Lawton, M.P. (1971). Personality traits in the mentally-impaired aged and their relationship to improvements in current functioning. Gerontologist, 11, 134-140.

Kuypers, J. (1969). Elderly persons en route to institutions: A study of changing perceptions of self and interpersonal relations. Unpublished doctoral dissertation, University of Chicago.

Larsen, E.B., Lo, B., Williams, N.E. (1986). Evaluation and care of elderly patients with dementia. J. Gen. Internal Med., 1, 116-126.

Lieberman, M.A., Prock, V., Tobin, S.S. (1968). Psychological effects of institutionalization. J. Gerontol., 23, 343-353.

Lieberman, M.A., Tobin, S.S. (1982). The Experience of Old Age: Stress, Coping, and Survival. New York: Basic Books.

Lindsley, O.R. (1964). Geriatric Behavioural Prosthetics. In Kastenbaum, R. (ed.). New Thoughts in Old Age. New York: Springer.

Lyons, W. (1982). Coping with cognitive impairment: some family dynamics and helping roles, J. Gerontol. Soc. Work, 4, 3-21.

Marchico-Greenfield (1986). C-O-N-N-E-C-T (Communication Need Not Ever Cease Totally): A communication enrichment project for families at the Jewish home and hospital for the aged. Unpublished paper.

Malzer, D.L., Cox C. (1987). A management program for ambulatory institutionalized patients with Alzheimer's disease and related disorders. Unpublished paper.

Pincus, M.A. (1968). Toward a Conceptual Framework for Studying Institutional Environments in Homes for the Aged. Unpublished Doctoral Dissertation, University of Wisconsin.

Pinkston, E.M., Levitt, J.L., Green, G.R., Linsk, N.L., Rzepnicki, T.L. (1982). Effective Social Work Practice. San Francisco: Jossey-Bass.

Reider, N. (1953). A type of transference to institutions. J. Hillside Hospital, 2, 23-29.

Rodin, J., Langer, E.J. (1977). Long-term effects of a control-relevant intervention within the institutionalized aged. J. Pers. Soc. Psychol., 35, 897-902.

Rosner, A. (1968). Stress and the maintenance of self-concept in the aged. Unpublished Doctoral Dissertation. The University of Chicago.

Safford, I. (1980). A program for families of the mentally impaired elderly. Gerontologist., 20, 656-60.

Safirstein, S. (1967). Institutional transference. Psychiat. Quart., 41, 557-566.

Smith, K.F., Bengtson, V.L. (1979). Positive consequences of institutionalization: solidarity between elderly parents and their middle-aged children. Gerontologist, 19, 438-447.

Tobin, S.S. (1972). The earliest memory as data for research. In Kent, D., Kastenbaum, R., Sherwood, S. (eds.). Research Planning and Action for the Elderly: Power and Potential of Social Science. New York: Behavioral Publications, 252-275.

Tobin, S.S. (1987). A structural approach to families. In Brubaker, T.H. (ed.). Aging, Health and Family. Newbury Park, CA.: Sage Publication, 42-55.

Tobin, S.S., Etigson, E.C. (1968). Effects of stress on the earliest memory. Arch. Gen. Psychiatry, 19, 436-444.

Tobin, S.S., Lieberman, M.A. (1976). Last Home for the Aged: Critical Implications of Institutionalization. San Francisco: Jossey-Bass.

Turner, B.F., Tobin, S.S., Lieberman, M.A. (1972). Personality Traits as predictors of institutional adaptation among the aged. J. Gerontol. , 27, 61-68.

Van Eck, L.A. (1972). Transference to the hospital. Psychoth. and Psychosom., 20, 135-138.

Vencente, L., Wiley, J.A., Carrington, R.A. (1979). The risk of institutionalization before death. Gerontologist., 19, 361-7.

Wilmer, H.A. (1962). Transference to a medical center. California Medicine, 96, 173-180.

CHAPTER 9

TELLING NEEDS FROM WISHES: A PRACTICAL AND INTEGRATED

APPROACH TO PSYCHIATRIC CARE OF THE ELDERLY

Adrian Grek, M.B., B. Ch., F.R.C.P.(C)
Queen St. Mental Health Centre and University of Toronto
Kenneth Shulman, M.D., F.R.C.P.(C)
Sunnybrook Medical Centre and University of Toronto
Toronto, Ontario

Other chapters in this book have described physical, psychological and social approaches to the mental complications of cerebral diseases in late life. A biopsychosocial synthesis is very alluring, but chimaeras may live more easily in compound words than in reality. The reconciliation of disparate forms of treatment is a formidable challenge, because it requires a realignment of priorities and resources which may threaten professional interests, prestige and relationships.

The needs of patients and their families must be distinguished from their fantasies and those of the attendant specialists. At some point, cure is the dream of every sick person, his family and his doctor. It is virtually never realized if the illness is the result of one of the degenerative cerebral processes of old age. Hope should not be abandoned, but if it is unrealistic, the bitterness and nihilism of failure will make the inevitable unbearable. The dismal plight of many dependent old people in even affluent societies graphically illustrates the failure of most contemporary approaches: life is long and the art short.

Take dementia as an example, although the same considerations might apply to other illnesses as well. The actual incidence of dementia is not known, but even if lower estimates are taken, say 0.6% per year over 65 (Schoenberg, Kokmen, Okazaki, 1987), 22,000 older Canadians may be faced with the spectre of losing their minds each year. Their first wish, and that of their families, might be that this were not happening, but of patients who present with "dementia for investigation", fewer than one in ten have something else (Larson, Reifler, Sumi, Canfield and Chinn, 1985). That being so, the next wish of the unfortunate majority might be that the dementia could be driven away, but fewer than one in a hundred of those in whom the diagnosis of dementia is established return to normal with treatment. In response to specific medical treatment, one quarter may improve intellectually for at least one month, and one eighth for at least one year. These improvements are likely to be seen only in those with specific clues in the history or on examination; less severe dementia; a short history; or a sudden deterioration (Larson, Reifler, Featherstone and English, 1984). And what of those - more than two thirds - in whom no cognitive improvement occurs? There is evidence that function autonomy and dignity can increase in a suitable environment (Edelson and Lyons, 1985). This could be considered the most common need of demented people. It is much less than cure, but it is far more than nothing.

Both cure and care have their price. Price is not the same as value, but when money is limited, it needs at least to be considered. To search for reversible causes of dementia in 22,000 people each year, making the use of the standard batteries suggested, would cost about $22 million a year. As mentioned, reversible factors are not often found; the commonest of them is polypharmacy, which can be detected without extensive investigation. Twenty-two million dollars may sound like a lot of money, but in Canada, it would pay for only about two to four days of basic nursing home care for the five to nine percent of people over 65 with moderate to severe dementia (Jeans, Helmes, Merskey, Robertson and Rand, 1987) who may need it. Basic nursing home care does not include the provision of an environment in which activity and independence can be flexibly encouraged. The cost of basic nursing home care is likely not very different from that of looking after a demented person at home. So although the yield of exhaustive routine investigation is very low, so is the *relative* cost, compared to the overall expenditure necessary.

[There are uncertainties about the rate of institutionalization, and the median survival after diagnosis.]

That cost is not the main issue may be reassuring to physicians who are traditionally uncomfortable with the view that it might be. There are, however, psychological and ethical aspects to consider as well. The dogged emphasis on identifying reversible factors may promote a spurious and cruel hope in the patient and the family, and postpone acknowledging and dealing with their day-to-day difficulties. Concentrating too hard on finding unlikely reversible factors may also have something to do with the well-known phenomenon of rejection by hospital doctors and consultants of patients if such a factor is not found. Without the possibility of a cure, it is as if nothing can be done. The sudden replacement of optimism by nihilism is neither fair nor correct, but is all too common. Such nihilism feeds on itself.

A patient abandoned to an unsatisfactory nursing home, or to the even
less satisfactory waiting list for an unsatisfactory nursing home, or left
to a spouse with insufficient resources to manage will become worse than
can simply be predicted from the stage of the disease. The response to
this decline may be as fragmented and ambivalent as the response to the
initial presentation, and a needless downward spiral may result.

Given the irreversible and progressive nature of the underlying illness
it is necessary to frame the therapeutic goals in terms other than cure.
"Excess disability" must be reduced; strengths and autonomy promoted as
much as is reasonable; respite provided to the families of patients; and
when institutionalization is really unavoidable, it should be dedicated to
activity and dignity as much as to convenience and cleanliness.

The system seems to do all it can to cure patients and keep them
alive, yet appears overwhelmed when they live too long. Technology fails
when it is needed least. The decisions about diagnostic tests, and
strategies for treatment and help for the family can be made on the basis
of a relatively straightforward but comprehensive history, observation,
and examination. This is not to deny the value of specialized knowledge
and skill, nor of the essential contributions of many disciplines, but
from a medical point of view, basic clinical practices and techniques must
not be sacrificed by specialists while others are acquired and developed.

If professional attitudes are flexible, there is a greater chance that
organizational structures can be developed to respond to the needs of
patients rather than the other way around. To a considerable extent, this
has been the experience of psychiatrists and geriatricians who have
developed services in Britain during the past twenty years (Arie, 1970;
Pitt, 1980; Glasscote, Guderman and Miles, 1977; Arie and Jolley, 1982;
Arie, 1986). It has been accepted that services must be comprehensive
rather than fragmented, and that they must be planned and developed in
response to the clearly identified needs of the population for whom they
are intended.

The identification of such needs has made clear the irrelevance to
psychogeriatrics of certain hallowed distinctions.

Firstly, the boundary between the hospital or clinic and the community
can be an obstruction. Patients must be assessed where they live in order
to obtain a proper perspective on their function at a stage early enough
to allow useful interventions.

Secondly, the peculiar constraints placed on psychiatrists primarily
engaged in fee-for-service office practice prevent ready adaptation to the

changing needs of elderly patients. A rigid schedule may prevent an
urgent home visit if required.

Thirdly, the rigid separation between individual sectors of service
does not serve this population well. Specialists, whether medically
trained or not, have to yield creatively and responsively to one another.
They must take an interest in matters beyond their traditional fields, and
yield "turf" and authority if they are not relevant to a particular
patient's circumstances. There has to be close collaboration between
psychiatric and medical services for it is meaningless to consider illness
in the elderly in either the physical or mental context without reference
to the other.

Similarly, the parallel and separate operation of "acute" and
"chronic" sectors is inappropriate. Acute services feel "stuck" with
"placement problems" and chronic institutions, isolated from the glamour,
feel abused, and do not feel compelled to respond quickly to the needs of
the acute care sector. As if the needs are those of the institutions
rather than the patient who becomes the victim of struggles among
professional groups for action and prestige! If the differentiation
between acute and chronic work is seen to be counter-productive there
might be no need for the struggles at all.

Finally, a sometimes unhelpful distinction is that between the patient
and the caregiver. The mental and physical well-being of caregivers, the
quality and nature of their relationship with an ill relative, and the
quality and extent of resources available to caregivers have all been
identified as factors very important in the outcome of mental illness in
the elderly (Rabins, 1982; Levin, Sinclair and Gorbach, 1983; Gilleard,
1984). Management at every level has to take both patient and caregiver
into account.

In Britain several innovations reflect the spirit and changing
practice necessary to meet the specific needs of this group of patients
and their families. Home assessment has already been mentioned and is the
mainstay of the evaluation. Day hospitals have been found to provide
relief for caregivers, and to delay institutionalization (Arie, 1979;
Greene and Timbury, 1979). A variant of the day hospital is the so-called
"travelling day hospital". Here, the professional expertise of the psychogeriatric team is brought to a variety of "day care" settings for a session
at a time. Assessment, consultation and appropriate intervention are
provided. This maximizes the use of the least intensive services. For
those frail old people who have trouble getting around, an alternative to
the day hospital has been a "sitting service" which sends paid "sitters"
to a patient's home to provide supervision for the patient and relief for
the caregiver (Rosenvinge, Guion and Dawson, 1986). Collaboration between

geriatric medical and psychiatric services is close in Britain ranging from individual consultations to the establishment of joint assessment units (Arie and Dunn, 1973; Pitt and Silver, 1980).

Such changes in attitudes and services must be rigorously evaluated to remain relevant and responsive. The complexity of the problems and resources make evaluation difficult. Randomized, double blind controlled studies of specific populations may be ethically and practically impossible. At this stage, it may be more important for services accurately and systematically to describe their experience while adhering to the principle of serving a clearly defined population. Sufficient numbers of descriptive surveys may help to develop an idea of the range and quantity of services, personnel and facilities necessary.

There are obviously difficulties inherent in these illnesses but there is also hope for better care. The British experience is encouraging, and so is the recent development of academic units in geriatric psychiatry in North America. Social pressures are forcing geriatrics into the mainstream of medicine and may help to change the direction of that stream. Medical and other professional schools will have to respond by training enthusiastic and skilled people who will ensure the relevance of their professions to the great challenge of the coming decades.

REFERENCES

Arie, T. (1970). The first year of the Goodmayes psychiatric service for old people. Lancet, 1179-1182.

Arie, T. (1979). Day Care in Geriatric Psychiatry. Age and Aging. Suppl. 8, 87-91.

Arie, T. (1986). Management of dementia: a review. Br. Med. Bull., 42, 91-96.

Arie, T., Dunn, T. (1973). A "do-it-yourself" psychiatric-geriatric unit. Lancet, 313-316.

Arie, T., Jolley, D. (1982). Making services work: organization and style of psychogeriatric services. In Levy, R., Post, F., (eds.). The Psychiatry of Late Life. Oxford, Blackwell, 222-251.

Edelson, J.S., Lyons, W.H. (1985). Institutional Care of The Mentally Impaired Elderly. New York: Van Nostrand Reinhold.

Gilleard, C.J. (1984). Living with Dementia. London: Croom Helm.

Glasscote, R.M., Guderman, J.E., Miles, D.E. (1977). Creative mental health services for the elderly. Washington, D.C., American Psychiatric Association.

Greene, J.G., Timbury, G.C. (1979). A geriatric psychiatry day hospital service: a five year review. Age and Ageing, 8, 49-53.

Jeans, E.R., Helmes, E., Merskey, H., Robertson, J.M., Rand, K.A. (1987). Some calculations on the prevalence of dementia in Canada. Can. J. Psychiatry, 32, 81-86.

Larson, E.B., Reifler, B.V., Featherstone, H.J., English, D.R. (1984). Dementia in elderly outpatients: a prospective study. Ann. Intern. Med., 100, 417-423.

Larson, E.B., Reifler, B.V., Sumi, S.M., Canfield, C.G., Chinn, N.M. (1985). Diagnostic evaluation of 200 elderly outpatients with suspected dementia. J. Gerontol., 40, 536-543.

Levin, E., Sinclair, J., Gorbach, P. (1983). The supporters of confused elderly persons at home. London: National Institute for Social Work.

Pitt, B. (1980). Growing points in the psychiatry of old age. Can. J. Psychiatry. 25, 1-25.

Pitt, B., Silver, C.P. (1980). The combined approach to geriatrics and psychiatry: Evaluation of a joint unit in a teaching hospital district. Age and Ageing, 9, 33-37.

Rabins, P.V. (1982). The impact of dementia on the family. JAMA, 248, 3, 333-335.

Rosenvinge, H., Guion, J., Dawson, J. (1986). Sitting service for the elderly confused. Health Trends, 18, 47.

Schoenberg, B.S., Kokmen, E., and Okazaki, H. (1987). Alzheimer's disease and other dementing illnesses in a defined United States population: incidence rates and clinical features. Ann. Neurol. 22, 724-729.

INDEX

Disinhibition, 5, 21, 72
Disorders, neuropsychiatric see
    Neuropsychiatric disor-
    ders
Disorganized thinking, 16, 17
Disorientation, 19
Disruptive behaviours see Beha-
    viour, disruptive
Distractibility, 6, 67
Distraction technique, 90-91
Dopamine, 9, 13, 56
Dopamine catabolism, 27
Dopamine decarboxylase, 13
Dopamine projections, 27
Dopamine-acetylcholine balance
    in Parkinson's disease, 9
Dopaminergic kindling, 27
Dopaminergic pathways, 9
Dorsal medial thalami, 8
Doxepin, 65
Dream content, 87
Drug interactions, 68
Drug-induced disorders, 53
Drugs, 62
    see also names of speci-
    fic drugs
DSM-III, 15, 16
DSM-III-R, 1, 16, 17, 18
Dysarthria, 25
Dysphoria, 14
Dysprosody, 21
Dysthymia, 59

Eating, 8
    see also Feeding
ECG see Electrocardiography
Echocardiography, 56
ECT see Electroconvulsive ther-
    apy
Education
    of caregivers, 163, 172-177
EEG see Electroencephalogram
EKG see Electrocardiography
Electrocardiography, 56, 65
Electroconvulsive therapy, 27

Electroencephalogram, 53
Emotion, 6, 9
    see also names of speci-
    fic emotions
Emotional lability, 6, 33, 35,
    71
Emotional life, subjective, 6
Empathetic rapport, 122-123,
    126, 128
Encephalitis, 26, 62, 67
Encephalitis, herpes, 19, 69, 70
Encephalopathy, hepatic, 63, 69,
    70
Encephalopathy, post-traumatic,
    74
Endocrine disorders, 2
    cause of dementia, 75
    cause of depression, 62, 63
    cause of organic anxiety
        syndrome, 20
    cause of organic delusional
        disorder, 69, 70
    cause of organic mood synd-
        rome, 20
Endogenous depression, 9
Environment
    sense of control over, 13
Environmental factors
    and behaviour, 160, 176, 178
    effect on patients with de-
        mentia, 175-176, 190
    quality of
        as a predictor of relocat-
            ion outcome, 170, 171
Ephedrine, 69, 70
Epilepsy, 2, 73
    cause of depression, 62, 63
    cause of organic delusional
        syndrome, 20, 69, 70
    cause of organic personality
        syndrome, 20, 71
Epilepsy, temporal lobe, 8
Ethical questions
    in behavioural therapy, 103-
        105